KU-319-840

Speech Therapy:
Principles and Practice

Betty Byers Brown

Senior Lecturer in Speech Pathology and Therapy, Department of Audiology and
Education of the Deaf, University of Manchester
Adviser on Speech Therapy to the Department of Health and Social Security

CHURCHILL LIVINGSTONE
EDINBURGH LONDON MELBOURNE AND NEW YORK 1981

CHURCHILL LIVINGSTONE
Medical Division of Longman Group Limited

Distributed in the United States of America by
Churchill Livingstone Inc., 19 West 44th Street, New
York, N.Y. 10036, and by associated companies,
branches and representatives throughout the world.

First published 1981

ISBN 0 443 02099 X

British Library Cataloguing in Publication Data
Brown, Betty Byers
    Speech therapy.
    1. Speech therapy
    I. Title
    616.85'506   RC423   80-41324

Printed in Singapore by Huntsmen Offset Printing Pte Ltd

Preface

It is incumbent upon every new generation of practitioners to make some statement about the state of the craft. Any attempt will be incomplete and will render the author vulnerable to adverse criticism from her contemporaries and subsequently from her successors. But we would not have learned our craft if previous speech therapists had not been willing to attempt some exposition of its principles and practice.

The expansion of speech therapy since the acceptance of the Quirk Report in 1972 has made the re-statement of its principles necessary but difficult. Common ground among the multiplicity of conditions which we now treat is difficult to find. But if we believe there is a specific discipline of speech therapy, a body of knowledge and consistent practice which is peculiar to ourselves, we must try to pass it on to our students.

This text contains many inconsistencies and some conventions which will seem outmoded. The inconsistencies, particularly with regard to terminology, to some extent represent our present position. Some out-moded conventions are purposely adopted in the absence of a better alternative. These include the term 'speech therapy' which, as the book purports to show, is not a helpful appellation for the range of work undertaken. The word 'patient' is not always suitable for the population served but is preferred to the word 'client' which is the only serious alternative. The male pronoun is used for the patient and the female for the therapist. This is because there are more male patients than female and more female therapists than male and the attempt to use alternatives is laborious and awkward.

The book is written at a time when speech therapy students are able to study their subject in the universities, polytechnics and colleges of education of Great Britain and are, therefore, exposed to a much wider range of information than was available to diploma students in speech therapy training schools. It is hoped that it may help them to find the core of their practice and that they will be able to use it as a springboard for their own discoveries.

Manchester,
1981

Betty Byers Brown

Acknowledgements

From a professional life singularly blessed by splendid colleagues it is only possible to mention those most directly concerned with this book.

Professor I.G. Taylor and the staff of the Department of Audiology and Education of the Deaf, University of Manchester, have welcomed and assisted the development of speech therapy in all its clinical and academic manifestations.

Elspeth McCartney has been extremely helpful in providing references and modern viewpoints.

Jennifer Warner, longtime friend and colleague, has continued to share her insights with me.

Ada Hindson has been of invaluable assistance with the manuscript. The Medical Illustration Department, University of Manchester, has turned my bird's nest into a useful diagram.

I am very much beholden to them all, as I am to my husband, David Jackson, for his unfailing faith and support.

B.B.B.

Contents

SECTION TWO Speech therapy in practice

Principles governing speech therapy

1

The nature of the work

It is a presumptuous deed to attempt to change the behaviour of other people and never more than when that behaviour is speech. Speech most indicates what we are and what we wish to be. It is the means by which we communicate with each other, express our thoughts and feelings and affirm our identity. Even when a person's speech is faulty or imperfect it may show understanding and expressiveness to a high degree.

So interference which seeks to make a change is only justified if the person is in need and the interference is reasonably calculated to help him. Since there are many children and adults who do experience severe difficulties in verbal communication, the profession of speech therapy has evolved. The most modest aim is to leave the person communicating more easily and effectively than he was before. His need is to be better understood and if therapy is successful he will be more intelligible, less adversely conspicuous and better accepted.

Speech therapy comprises a variety of forms of speech and language intervention, guidance and support. Since speech is the preferred method of communication in our society, those who cannot use it easily are handicapped. For most of us speech, in the sense of spoken language, is a convenient, flexible, and straightforward way of conveying information or exchanging thoughts and feelings. For the unfortunate exceptions speech therapy exists to amend and develop the means by which language is conveyed. It seeks to help people understand and use conventional forms of language. If this is not possible the less conventional forms must be explored. For speech therapy is concerned with the very stuff of language, the use of any symbol system to reveal thought and to share that thought with others.

The act of speech is successful as communication when it is understood and acted upon by others. If a speaker cannot make himself understood the fault may lie in the way his words are uttered or the way in which his thoughts are formulated. A listener who shares the same language background as the speaker expects to be able to understand him. He will usually make some attempt to worry out a message that is imperfectly conveyed by using the context of that message. If the speaker is familiar to him he will draw upon knowledge of that speaker's characteristic behaviour. Listeners vary in their ability to adapt themselves to the unusual. Most of us can become very good at understanding one other person; a child whose speech is immature and whose thoughts are developing; a husband or father whose established language has been disrupted; a friend whose speech idiosyncrasies have become familiar. However to understand all speakers whose performance differs from mature, conventional standards demands a high degree of dedicated training and natural aptitude.

The first attribute of a speech therapist must be the ability to observe and interpret language behaviour. The interpretations will encompass the embryonic speech signals of the handicapped infant and the complete but deviant system of the older person whose speech has been acquired abnormally. They will also extend to the fragments of language offered by those whose skills have been pathologically disrupted. All courses of study offered to speech therapy students equip them to observe and interpret. But they can only perfect these attributes if they have the innate qualities of warmth and responsiveness. Listening is a skill and listening to abnormal speech demands a high degree of sympathy and creativity. While scientific analysis will be required to establish the nature of the speech difficulty, it will not draw forth the communication in the first place. It is the relationship between therapist and patient which allows the whole process of observation, deduction, analysis and treatment to be carried through. It is this that sustains the interest and will on both sides and makes a common venture out of a demanding task.

The speech therapist is not alone in caring for the speech handicapped. The process of identifying and treating all manner of verbal disorders contains elements which can be more properly carried out by members of other professions. But the speech therapist must be acquainted with every aspect of the process, and be able to see it through from start to finish. She must know the point at which the patient may be helped more by other people and must see that he is put in the way of this help. She will be involved in an integrated series of activities which should lead from the initial identification of the speech handicapped and dependent person to the establishing of his independence in language use.

Emphasis has always been placed by the speech therapy profession upon the personal qualities of its members. This emphasis is well justified by the nature of the work in which they are engaged. But the work also demands minds trained to grasp relationships and trace connections. It exists to solve problems and its success will be measured by its effectiveness in doing so. For the problem to be solved its essential elements must be recognised: this is assessment. Sometimes the picture is such that the element which is at fault can be identified and named or described: this is diagnosis. Both assessment and diagnosis are part of the therapeutic process and both should lead to the working out of treatment. An assessment is an estimate of the present position based on scrutiny of all available information. A diagnosis is a formal statement of the nature of the cause. These words are sometimes used interchangeably but they should not be for they stand for different things. Both are necessary for full understanding of the condition but it may not be possible to achieve both before treatment is started. Treatment may legitimately be undertaken to test out a hypothetical cause or to provide a further aspect of assessment.

It is helpful to retain the idea of therapy as hypothesis testing even if the condition has been diagnosed with some assurance. There is always the question of how far a cause can account for the symptom presented, particularly when the symptom is a disorder of speech, itself a complicated and compound skill. If speech impairment is present there will be a discrepancy between the speaker's attempts and society's demands. Speech therapy exists to render this discrepancy less handicapping and it must therefore be constantly concerned with the nature of the attempt and the nature of the need. It will be based on understanding of what speech is and of the developmental process by which it is acquired. It can only succeed if it arises from knowledge of the communicative system of society and the needs of the particular person who is failing to use the system.

There are several ways in which speech can be studied and speech breakdown explored. It is helpful to consider models of procedure developed by doctors, psychologists and linguists. Much of our therapeutic method has been based on such models but the individual therapist does not always formulate the steps she is taking hence the process may not be clear to the less experienced. A model of procedure gives direction and ensures that nothing of significance is overlooked. It must always be combined with the case history compiled from information given by the patient and his family.

THE MEDICAL MODEL

This method of procedure starts by observing the symptom and then seeks to trace it to a cause. It attempts to identify any disease or physical abnormality and then to consider the extent to which this can account for the symptom. From identification of the disease process it will move to consideration of attitude or environment. Physical examination is an essential part of the procedure.

The clinician working in this way will consider all the factors that are known to be strongly associated with this particular symptom. If none of them is present she will extend her search towards more obscure or more deviously connected factors. The less experienced clinician will cast her net widely in the hope that something significant may be found. The skilled practitioner however will work deductively and economically, using one set of results to tell her what the next move should be and only exposing her patient to as many tests as are essential to reveal the nature of the complaint. This may be illustrated by the following:

Child 3 years
Presenting symptom = Unintelligible speech
Major known causes = Hearing loss
                            Mental retardation
As these two major factors are vital to the child's whole development they must first be explored.

Hearing loss
  Known or suspected correlates:
    Genetic determinants
    Familial incidence
    Maternal illness/infection (rubella)
    Prematurity
    Anoxia
    Infectious disease
    Structural abnormality
    Otitis media.
  Indications:
    Abnormal response to sound
    Limited babbling
    Delay in speech onset
    Frustrations and temper
    Tantrums.

Hearing test Suspicion confirmed or negated by audiological assessment.

Mental retardation
  Known or suspected correlates:
    Genetic determinants
    Familial incidence
    Maternal illness/infection (rubella)
    Prematurity
    Anoxia
    Brain damage or disease.
  Indications:
    Delayed milestones
    Immaturity
    Hypotonia.

In the absence of hearing loss and presence of several of the factors listed, mental retardation is a strong possibility and may be confirmed or negated by psychological assessment and by general paediatric and specific medical investigation. The speech therapist will proceed in the same way, concentrating her observations upon the child's language and associating her findings with those of the doctor, psychologist and audiologist.

Child 3 years
Known correlates of hearing loss and mental retardation as already listed and also:

Hearing loss
  Language indications
    Absence of H/F sounds
    Absence of unstressed sounds
    Imitation improved by visual model.
Mental retardation
  Language indications
    Generally immature phonology
    Generally immature syntax
    Poor attention to speech detail.

The same procedure will be carried out with adults who have noticed a change in speech.

Adult 65 years
Presenting symptom = Slurred speech

Major known causes = Cerebrovascular accident. (c.v.a.)
Neurological disease

The key to this diagnosis would lie in the medical case history and neurological examination. Early distinction would be made between peripheral and central speech function. The former may be associated with *motor neurone* disease which would be revealed by examination of muscle tone and other neurological features. It may also be associated with *upper motor neurone* lesions involving both pyramidal tracts. In these cases a more careful distinction must be made between:

An/ *An/* *An/*
Dysarthria *Dyspraxia* *Dysphasia*

necessitating examination of muscle tone, involuntary and voluntary movement and cognitive/linguistic function.

The speech therapist would be interested in the following factors:

Control of speech organs in chewing, swallowing and speech.

Phonation Articulatory agility

Pitch Volume Word finding

Nasality Discourse

In the absence of clear neurological guidance the patient's performance would allow a differential diagnosis to be put forward.

Investigations along medical lines are extremely valuable and frequently vital in speech therapy but they do have disadvantages. One is that attention is very much focused upon the cause of the condition. This may delay attempts to make life easier for everyone and hold up treatment. It is not always profitable to spend much time trying to decide on a precise factor underlying a symptom. In young, developing children it may not be possible to isolate any one causal factor. The position may be one of developmental vulnerability which circumstance or mismanagement has turned into handicap. In such cases it is very much more helpful to alleviate anxiety by improving communication than to prolong it by protracted investigation. There is always the danger too of iatrogenic malfunction where the investigations themselves introduce the idea of disease. With young children the speech therapist may find her best guidance from a developmental model.

THE DEVELOPMENTAL MODEL

Normal children move through stages of development in more or less the same way and acquire skills at more or less the same time. These stages and skills are well documented and the outside limits of normality delineated. A child whose development in any area is causing concern may be placed within this framework and his progress charted. A developmental profile can be drawn up which will show whether the discrepancies between his skills and other children's are so considerable as to suggest abnormality. It will also show the child's strengths and weaknesses; the areas where he is up to average and those in which he falls short. The skilled clinician will be able to decide from such a profile whether to investigate further and also how to give guidance.

The following illustration is a *Developmental profile* of a little girl referred because the medical officer strongly suggested deafness. Her age on referral was 23 months and the following notes were made at 25 months. Looking at this cursory record we can see that the child was up to average or slightly ahead during her early development and the only significant delay is in speech. Hearing would certainly be the first target for investigation, however this proved to be normal. The child was taken under observation and her comprehension assessed at intervals. A parent guidance programme and language stimulation was subsequently required. Although in the majority of cases such a delay would not be abnormal, in this case it was significant and the child needed help.

Skill	Age	Normal range
Sucking	From birth	√
Chewing	All foods now chewed (25 months)	√
Sitting (unsupported)	6 months	√ (early)
Walking alone	12 months	√ (early)
Feeding herself	22 months	√
Clean (day) (night)	24 months	not yet outside normal range
Dry (day)	—	not yet outside normal range
(night)	—	not yet outside normal range
First words	—	×
First sentences	—	×

Too heavy a reliance upon a developmental model will also have disadvantages. There is a very wide range of variation within normal development and exactitude of recording must vary with the skill under observation. It is much easier to observe and thence to note change in motor functions where something can be seen to be happening than in the perceptive and cognitive skills where everything is going on inside the infant. There is considerable danger of over interpretation by parents and therapists when cognitive behaviour is being studied and recorded anecdotally as distinct from experimentally.

There is also the possibility of being too concerned about delays and traits of development in one child because the whole family and its history is not known to the therapist. A doctor or a teacher who has seen many members of one family will frequently have a more relaxed attitude towards individual behaviour than a speech therapist who may only see the one. A balanced attitude will however emerge from increased experience. Careful study of normal development is now a bedrock of clinical practice and therefore of student training also. We now need to take much more cognisance of very early, pre-speech behaviour, and know how to build this into our developmental profiles. Much of our observation is still too broad to be useful as a treatment guide for the severely handicapped.

There is no need to keep separate these two models of investigation and indeed they are most effective when used in combination. As has been stated, the developmental profile will suggest the need for deeper investigation and once a medical investigation has been carried out progress may be charted developmentally. The experienced clinician moves from one method to another checking and recording. Her findings will be put into an increasingly rich matrix of knowledge and observation. The less experienced therapist will work a little more doggedly and laboriously until she becomes used to the implications of her results.

There are many patients for whom a developmental model is not appropriate but where medical procedure is not entirely satisfactory either. In these cases it is helpful to generate another procedure based on language theory. This model may also be used to provide a check on procedure generated by other models.

THE LANGUAGE MODEL

Normal use of language has been shown to involve a number of physical and psychological processes which may be depicted diagrammatically. Representation can be made of the properties themselves and of the way that their function is regulated and controlled. If an individual person's language behaviour is plotted against such a representation any weak links will be revealed. The presence or absence of all the component parts should be apparent and also the mechanism's capacity for control (Fig. 1).

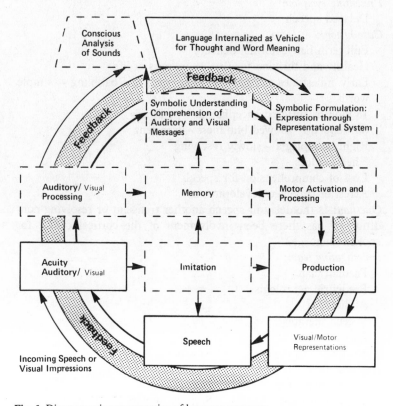

Fig. 1 Diagrammatic representation of language processes

Once this representation is made hypotheses may be advanced to account for what is happening or failing to happen. Experiments can then be devised which will test out the hypotheses and at the same time indicate remedy. Many of our current tests for aphasia are based upon a theoretical language model, as are treatment measures designed to promote fluency or regulate utterance. If no hard evidence is available as to what is actually happening the therapist must temporarily abandon the search for a cause and venture forth upon the basis of a reasonable hypothesis. In order to prevent too many random ventures of this kind the theoretical framework should be clearly drawn up. This will provide the necessary checks and possibly illumination also. The following case illustrates how all three approaches may be combined:

Boy of 2 years 8 months.
Presenting symptom:
    Delayed speech
Case history:
    Full term baby, normal delivery
    Healthy and thriving for first 18 months of life
    Early milestones normal including speech – babbling – simple words
    18 months suffered encephalitic type illness
    Subsequently showed blindness – transient
    Right hemiplegia – slowly resolving
    ? hearing loss
    Loss of comprehension for speech
    Arrest of language development.
Question: Is the delay in speech another transient or resolving condition or has there been involvement of the cortical centre for spoken language?
Investigating team:
    Paediatrician
    Paediatric neurologist
    Audiologist
    Speech therapist
    Psychologist.

Medical investigations	*Results*
Motor function	
Muscular tone	Normal
Co-ordination	Slightly impaired
Involuntary movement	Absent
Cranial nerves	Intact
Vision	Within normal limits (as far as could be ascertained)
Hearing	Within normal limits as tested by distraction testing and impedance audiometry
Sensation	Within normal limits (so far as could be ascertained).

Speech investigation
  Motor functions
    Tongue
    Lips   } Normal
    Palate

Vocalising	Present; tone slightly nasal
Prosodic features	Present; variations of pitch and volume, also duration
Phonetic inventory	Limited to nasals, simple plosives and vowels
Words	Very few present in utterance; comprehension of simple words present
Sentences	Not used; simple sentences comprehended.

  Cerebral function

Attention	Disturbed; highly distractible
Laterality	Undecided
Play	Stereotyped and repetitive; lack of symbolic play.

Developmental assessment

Locomotion	Approximately 2 year level
Play	18 months ⟶ 2 years
Care of self	Approximately 2½ years
Social responses	Appropriate for age level
Language	Symbolic understanding – 2 year level
	Verbal comprehension – 2 year level
	Speech (verbal expression) 18 months level.

Neither the medical nor the development information led to a definitive diagnosis of aphasia as distinct from language delay or mild mental retardation. These therefore remained as hypotheses to be tested by response to treatment and parent guidance.

Hypothesis 1: Delayed language
  Management: Parent guidance and therapy comprising:
    1. Attention training
    2. Auditory training
    3. Vocabulary building
    4. Directed play
    5. Speech stimulation and reinforcement.

Commenced at 3 years

Prediction: Good response to therapeutic measures = accelerated language growth: improvement should be discernable in 3 months. Child should show greater linguistic growth than could be accounted for by maturation when re-asssessed in 6 months and 12 months.

Hypothesis 2: Mental retardation

Management: As for hypothesis 1

Prediction: Slow growth in all areas: some slight improvement sustained over period of 6 months. Child develops at a rate commensurate with, or slightly below maturation and thus shows essentially the same picture when re-tested at 6 and 12 monthly intervals.

Hypothesis 3: Aphasia

Management: As for hypothesis 1

Prediction: Slow response to attention training = very slow growth in language; severe delay in moving into 2-word sentences; child shows greater improvement in non-verbal than verbal skills but is easily confused and erratic in his responses. Re-assessment at 6 monthly intervals shows increased discrepancy between non-verbal and verbal attainments.

In this case hypothesis 3 was confirmed. At the age of 3 years 8 months simple two-word utterances were established as a regular feature but distractability was still a marked feature. Consideration was given to future needs and the following recommendations made:

1. Continue language therapy and parent guidance
2. Recommend language unit placement at school entry.
3. Continue regular psychological assessments.

These recommendations were prepared for continuing language handicap having regard also to the possibility of transfer of dominance and development of the speech centre on the right side of the brain. Therefore also

4. Continue regular paediatric/neurological examinations.

At this point the child's condition can be assessed against the *language model* and this used as a continuing guide in therapy.

Areas of weakness would be carefully noted and effort made to strengthen them through associated skills. Thus language processing, comprehension and expression through the use of symbols would continue to be targets of therapy for this child. Continuous attention would be given to strengthening feedback and memory.

The case history

Any investigatory procedure will be experimental and many will be inappropriate if they are not related to the individual case history. This must be compiled by the speech therapist though the range of her enquiry as well as its focus will depend upon what has gone before. Sometimes a patient will be referred when many investigations have already been carried out and much information compiled. Sometimes there is barely more than the patient's name, age and a comment upon his lack of speech. Since the Quirk Committee supported a more open system of referral, the speech therapist sees adults and children who may not have received medical examination. It is therefore incumbent upon her to be highly alert to the need for medical opinion. The following shows how the speech therapist will gear her case history taking to complete the picture.

Case history 1

Peter, aged 7 years 4 months was referred for investigation by the school medical officer because of stammering and possible language disorder.

Family	3rd child and 1st son of healthy parents. Both older sisters had developmental speech difficulties
Ante-natal and birth history	Normal. Child weighed 9 lbs; normal colour, cried and sucked normally
Post-natal	Uneventful; continued to thrive
Milestones	Early milestones passed at the normal age
Walking	Noted as late by mother in comparison with both older sisters. No actual date recorded
Toilet training	Normal age
Feeding and self-help	Normal. No divergence from average developmental pattern observed
Temperament	Placid and independent
Hand skills	Rather late in developing hand preference. Some clumsiness in evidence from 3 years onwards. Now uses left hand but still has difficulty in writing and drawing neatly
Speech	First words rather late compared with average but not markedly so. Attempts at early words not clear but intelligible to mother. Very late in joining words. Sentences not used regularly until around 3

	years. Speech never clear. Comprehension seemed good. Present speech pattern frequently incoherent with some stammering
Education	Entered nursery and infant class at normal age. Speech still delayed but did not prevent good adaptation. Subsequently teachers became concerned because of slow growth of language and poor hand control
Motor development	Initially normal but recently Peter has been conspicuous among his peers for clumsiness and poor sense of rhythm and movement
Intelligence	Low average on psychological tests but this 'is almost certainly an underestimate' because the boy was penalised by the verbal component and by slowness on motor tasks.

This history immediately opens up areas for investigation. While auditory acuity needs to be checked it is unlikely to be the major faulty factor in the development. In Peter's case acuity was normal. The main diagnostic area is that of psycho-linguistic function. The history suggests a disorder of the kind described in the early literature as *central language imbalance* or *cluttering* and now usually discussed under *development dysphasia*. This condition has a possible genetic basis and if so usually involves more than one member of the family though the manifestation may be different.

With the picture of clumsiness and delayed speech the whole area of sequential movement and patterning merits investigation. Speech/language investigations must therefore focus on sound and word sequences; phonology and syntax; narrative skills and word finding. The stammer or non-fluency should first be investigated in relation to possible language inadequacy and sequencing and co-ordination difficulties.

Psychological assessment should concentrate on visual perception and eye-motor co-ordination; also motor-spatial perception. From these combined investigations into visual, auditory and motor processing a profile of strengths and weaknesses should emerge which can provide the basis for therapy and remedial teaching.

Case history 2
Mrs A. aged 36 years was referred for investigation and treatment of voice loss. This had occurred several times during the last 2 years.

Occupation   Housewife
Family situation Married with three children aged 10, 7 and 5. All healthy and presenting no problems. Husband in good health, loving and supportive. No family problems or financial difficulties.
Health history   Good. No recent illnesses or accidents
Inheritance   Both parents alive and well. No history of emotional disorders or neurological disease
Examinations   1. Laryngological: Vocal cords slightly reddened but moving well. No disease process apparent. Cough normal; full vocal cord approximation.
                  2. Hearing: Normal acuity.

Patient has not reached menopause and reports no significant voice change associated with menstruation.

History of vocal disorder. First experienced voice loss following amateur theatricals at local church. Patient active in the organisation of the performances as well as playing leading role. Subsequently has noticed vocal fatigue following choir rehearsal and theatricals. Voice usually returns to normal some two to three days following performance. Intermittent periods of vocal fatigue recalled during the last three or four years but no sustained voice loss until recently.

This history obviously suggests some additional burden imposed on the voice which it cannot meet. As vocal dysfunction is frequently associated with a combination of emotional as well as purely vocal factors, investigation would explore any particular stresses and anxieties associated with speech and singing. It would then explore the actual conditions in which performances were given and see whether the patient was equipped to use her voice in such conditions. Therapy would almost certainly concentrate on vocal re-training and psychological support.

In both these histories there are possible interpretations relying entirely on psychological/emotional grounds. With the boy a case could be made out for stammering as a protest against the dominance or extreme competition of two older sisters. With the woman the onus could immediately be placed upon the husband/wife relationship or the lack of personal satisfaction through the domestic role. Both interpretations may eventually prove true, but in the first instance it is wisest to work through the organic, habitual and learning factors and test these out before moving too strongly into the field of neuroses. By this route both therapist and patient may be assured that nothing has been overlooked and any diagnosis of emotional/psychological disorder will be arrived at after due deliberation and deduction.

Speech therapy is fundamentally a case centred science. It is from the intensive study of individual cases that it derives its strengths and insights. This does not mean that all treatment has to be completely new-minted. There are many common features in language handicap and it is because of these that treatment measures can be advised and their effects predicted. The extent to which any method is useful to more than the one individual served depends upon the way in which it has been constructed. If it is based upon principles of language function it should be generally applicable and transferable. The success of speech therapy is not only dependent upon individual care but upon the extent to which the therapist can work within the framework of ideas and conventions which govern the acquisition and use of language in society.

2

The nature of the skills

Consideration of the nature of speech therapy inevitably leads from description of the task to delineation of the skills required to carry out the task. They are far from easy to separate. The therapist is trying to produce a change in the direction of normal communication. At the very least the patient must be left a little better off than he was before. The improvement may be in his accomplishment, his attitude or his insight, but it must occur. There is no justification for the time and expense of professional intervention if the patient does not derive some benefit that he could not gain elsewhere. There is no justification for demanding the skilled attention of the speech therapist unless she can bring some care which is precisely relevant to the need.

If the first attribute of the speech therapist is her ability to observe and interpret language behaviour, the second must be a disciplined sensitivity to other people's needs. This sensitivity will dictate the timing of therapeutic intervention as well as its nature. Therapy is a continuous and dynamic interchange between the people concerned. It moves swiftly from broad considerations to detailed study. It must maintain control of the whole while concentrating on a part. The essential aim of improved communication must be combined with close attention to the improvement of small sub-skills like sound discrimination and production.

A third attribute is resource. Speech therapy contains many procedures which have been shown to be effective and which are sturdily rooted in observation and theory, but it contains few fully developed techniques which have been systematically charted and have proved to be invariably efficacious. There have not been enough studies of treatment efficacy to allow speech therapists to quote results with confidence, and so the clinician must select the most suitable procedure rather than seek an invariable remedy. She must devise the best way to bring about the necessary change by logical as well as by imaginative steps. The greater her knowledge of speech and other manifestations of language the more possibilities she can command.

Although effective speech has been described as an economical way of communicating it is also very rich and complex in nature. It contains a very large number of elements, many of which can be called upon to compensate for weakness in another. A skilled speaker uses a whole range of emphasis, tone colour, intonation and pronunciation to give character and clarity. He will select his words with care so that they convey his thoughts adequately and then underline the flavour of those thoughts by clear and vivid expositon. The greater his skill, the more possibilities are open to him. He may speak elaborately or succinctly but his speech will be suitable to its content and the occasion. He may employ idiosyncratic expressions or unusual emphases but only to serve a particular purpose. Such speech is interesting to listen to and commands attention.

Poor speech may be halting, monotonous, displeasing to the ear and limited or stereotyped in content. As such it will not command the listener's attention. It must be distinguished from that abnormal speech which is prevented by physical or psychological factors from conveying its messages adequately. This distinction is always made by speech therapists who are well aware that their province is with the second group and not the first. In making the distinction some points are however lost. The speech background and family standard is a highly important element in language stimulation or re-habilitation. A poor speaker with limited verbal ability who has suffered voice loss or dysphasia is much more restricted in his expressivity than one who has the same degree of loss but who previously had been able to exploit and take pleasure in the whole speech process. If the latter can master the emotional shock of his initial loss he will find plenty of speech components still left which he will learn to use skillfully, using a warm tone to help out a sparse expression or an increase of volume to replace a former variation of speed.

Even a child who has not attained fluent speech will show at an early stage whether he enjoys word selection and likes to experiment. The speech therapist must share this pleasure with him and encourage his individual mastery over the process in a manner which is personal as well as conventional. With logical and analytical approaches to treatment now current there is some danger that the fun and creativity is going of individual therapy. This is sad and could be self-defeating.

The speech therapist must be able to perceive how individual people want to express themselves; the value they place on speech and the kind of language they share with their families. She must use the same enjoyable language in her therapy. We all speak more easily to people with whom we expect to share the same language environment. The expression 'who speaks my language' covers attitude and sympathy as much as forms of words. If any patient has to add to his communication difficulties the onus of having to express himself to his therapist as a stranger, he will make little progress in speaking for himself. When any such onus is added it should be part of the therapeutic programme to expand the patient's skill, not an accidentally imposed hurdle.

There will of course be many instances where the patient's natural language cannot be the main target of therapy. He may have to be taught a more formal, circumscribed means because he remains unable to deduce the essential elements from the language round about him or to generate the process for himself. Even when she teaches an apparently artificial method of speech production or fluency control the therapist will judge her success by the command her patient gains over this utterance and the extent to which he can make it his own. For much of her work though she will rely upon stimulating her patients to experiment so that they have the pleasure of gaining control over the rules of language and using them creatively.

The question of the therapist's own speech has become a slightly vexed one. At one time it was required to provide the best possible model and much time was therefore spent by the student clinician on improving her speech. Now the onus is much more on general communicative ability using colloquial forms and informal utterance as seems appropriate. But however much she subscribes to utilitarian rather than aesthetic criteria the speech therapist still has to be able to demonstrate a wide range of vocal and verbal behaviour. She may be called upon to rehabilitate the voice of an opera singer or the language of a man of letters as well as the child with articulatory difficulties. She must have command over any individual consonant and vowel and also be able to regulate her fluency and change her tone immediately and accurately. So her own speech must remain her best equipment and needs the maintenance demanded by any other piece of equipment. It is her livelihood and her advertisement.

The speech therapist must combine the qualities of sympathy and flexibility with a clear sense of purpose. She must know what to do and how to do it. She must also know how she has achieved any results that have come about during therapy. This is not to suggest that the results have been achieved entirely by her efforts, nor is it to remove from her that much prized attribute of clinical intuition. It is rather to put such intuition into its proper place as servant not master. There is nothing magical about therapy but there are judgements that arise from tacit knowing as well as objective experience. During therapy the clinician will constantly adjust her tactics or modify her procedures as the result of tiny, almost imperceptible clues that she receives subliminally as well as through conscious observation. She must check and re-examine her procedures carefully and critically if she is to command them.

It is wise to train oneself from the beginning to analyse a task and deduce which of its components is most important. Then in retrospect one may consider whether the intervention provided was in fact helpful and if so why. The clinician who is too often surprised by success is one who is not developing her clinical judgement. It need hardly be said that the same thing is true of the clinician who is constantly surprised by failure.

Plans of action must be drawn up, considered and modified. The process starts with identification, moves on to assessment and diagnosis and thence to a logically derived treatment procedure and considered prognosis. Modifications are made as new evidence appears or as changes take place. If too great a modification has to be made it suggests that the initial plan was too hastily assembled or ill-advised. None of us however are gifted with such prescience that we can devise a once and for all plan covering every contingency. Indeed to assume that this were possible would be to rob therapy of one of its great delights; the gradual emergence of the patient as creator of his own aid.

The experienced clinician works as efficiently in treatment as she does in diagnosis, moving from one procedure to another, matching, checking and discarding. This is because she has built up a clinical memory comprised of persons and procedures. Recollection of one small boy may come to the help of another; success in monitoring fluency by one method may prompt its use in a similar case. Her efficiency is also much increased by what her experience tells her she can leave out. An oral inspection may not be necessary for a young child whose chewing is normal and whose speech is clear even if his language is delayed, but it will be vital if the speech is slightly nasal and there is more than average dribbling. The inexperienced clinician is wise to move more slowly, checking all relevant items as she goes, as otherwise the procedure she skips will be the one that contained the most vital piece of information.

Whatever her degree of experience and whatever the manner in which she works there will be skilled activities which every therapist must employ at some time. We are what we do and professional identity arises from the kinds of activities that we carry out. We are loth to itemise them for fear that they become fixed and fossilised or that our students are then trained to work mechanically rather than logically and creatively. Divorced from its clinical matrix, a list of tasks appears bald and finite. It also serves the image of a mendicant with his bag of tricks rather than the scientific image to which we aspire. Even so, the established practice of a speech therapist will include general and specific activities which can be listed.

General and abiding
The speech therapist should always be prepared to give support, guidance and counsel; the attributes that mark a caring profession. She must also be able to demonstrate the standards of voice, speech, language and fluency which are her professional equipment and show others how they may be attained. She must always be able to promote language use and teach language structure.

Particular and selective
1. Modifying behaviour
2. Training attention
3. Training listening
4. Training auditory discrimination and judgement
5. Training movement
6. Teaching control over patterns of movement
7. Teaching sequential skills
8. Training imitation
9. Teaching sound production
10. Developing vocabulary
11. Teaching representational systems of expression
12. Teaching relaxation and control of posture.

These activities can be considered within different frameworks. They can be seen as building in attributes of normal development missed by handicapped children.

Training focus or skill	Normal development
Modifying behaviour	Occurs throughout childhood in response to parental reward and punishment subsequently re-inforced or negated by environment

Training focus or skill	Normal development
Attention	Starts in infancy and moves through stages of distractability and rigidity in the early years; thence becomes single-channelled and then dual channelled; is normally well controlled by school entry level (Cooper et al, 1978)
Listening	Can be trained from early infancy, based upon normal acuity and assisted by development of attention; developed by reward and sustained by interest
Auditory discrimination and judgement	Ability to discriminate can be demonstrated in early infancy; used actively as child discovers speech units; provides the basis for linguistic growth
Movements	At first reflex; gradually become selective and controlled; practice leads to automatic movement at some levels and in others to improved range and precision
Control over patterns of movement	Feature of neuro-muscular maturation and cerebral dominance
Sequential skills	Acquired through visual, auditory and motor-sensory modalities as a feature of normal learning; associated with neurological maturation and cerebral dominance
Imitation	Normal activity in first 2–3 years of life in the presence of an attractive or vivid model; linguistically it shows the child testing the hypotheses he has formed about the nature of language
Sound production	Vocalising; babbling; subsequently sounds used as 'anchor points' to manipulate other linguistic features
Vocabulary	Learned from parents and others in infant environment and then more formally extended by teacher notably through reading
Representational systems	First worked out in play during second year of life and subsequently shown in language; associated with conceptual development
Relaxation and control of posture	The ability to relax is present throughout childhood unless interfered with by anxiety; control of posture emerges during the infant years starting with head control; it may be disrupted, temporarily by growth spurts

Children will also make use of transitory skills such as gesture which the therapist may train as a compensatory activity in the handicapped.

The same activities can be employed therapeutically in cases of communication breakdown.

Training focus or skill	Condition	Purpose of training
Modifying behaviour	Stammering Vocal dysfunction Language disorder	Replace present behaviour with something more propitious or effective
Attention	Language delays and disorders Acquired aphasia	Create or restore attribute affected by brain damage

Training focus or skill	Condition	Purpose of training
Attention	Stammering	Reduce self preoccupation and improve objectivity
Listening	Dysphasia Stammering Vocal dysfunction	Improve self-monitoring following recognition of standard
Auditory discrimination and judgement	All conditions	Match utterance to a model and then to self-correct
Movements	A/dysarthria A/dyspraxia A/dyspraxia	Train or re-train a pattern nearer to the normal and to develop kinaesthetic memory
Control over movement patterns	All cases of neuro-muscular disability including dysarthria Dyspraxia Vocal dysfunction Stammering	Establish or re-establish control where disability has interrupted flow of movement
Sequential skills	Aphasia Cluttering	Teach or re-create structure and establish monitoring
Imitation	All conditions	Offer contrasting and correct activity to that performed abnormally
Sound production	Anarthria Aphonia Apraxia Articulatory or phonetic disorder	Promote ability to initiate and control individual sounds and sound combinations
Vocabulary	Language delay Dysphasia Cluttering	Assist recall and retention and to improve exactitude in verbal expression
Representational systems (non-verbal) (verbal)	Aphasia Anarthria As above and in all forms of language disability	Present alternatives to verbal communication Promote verbal communication
Relaxation and control of posture	Stammering Vocal dysfunction	Reduce interference and distortion and promote ease

In the case of the little boy used in illustration in Chapter 1 the following skills were emphasised.

Training focus or skill	State of development	Purpose of training
Attention	Interrupted by illness; regressed to stages 1 and 2	Restore essential basis for learning
Listening	Affected by above	Assist language growth

Training focus or skill	State of development	Purpose of training
Sequential skills	Impaired by neurological insult	Teach structure
Imitation	Fleetingly present, needing useful application.	Promote play and verbal activity
Vocabulary	Approximately 12 months retarded	Necessary tool of expression and understanding
Representational systems	Approximately 12 months retarded	Develop play and thence language

The tasks listed as being the rightful remit of the speech thera-pist do not of course represent the entire range or summation of her role, but they are all areas in which she must be competent if she is to offer herself as a professional worker on behalf of the speech handicapped. Students are therefore trained to carry out such tasks during their clinical apprenticeship. When properly combined with a theoretical background to the conditions comprehended in com-munication breakdown, they will equip the graduating speech therapist to start her clinical career. As that career progresses her increased familiarity with the many manifestations of communica-tion breakdown and her increased experience in many aspects of human relations, will enlarge her clinical repertoire.

There are many areas into which speech therapists may now ven-ture with some degree of assurance. Some will prefer the prophylactic field and spend most time working with parents or nursery teachers. Others will develop a taste for measurement and will concentrate on specialised assessments. Some will become con-vinced of the importance of psychotherapeutic techniques and may become further qualified in this area. Others will be drawn to work with the deaf and may develop special interest in visual display systems allied to language training. These interests will often emerge during the student period and indeed before this, thus dic-tating the choice of course for which the student applies.

When the unified profession of speech therapy was formed in this country with the creation of the College of Speech Therapists in 1945, it was the intention that all speech therapists should come into the profession through the College's Examination for the Dip-loma. The course of events which lead to revision of the decision is fully charted in the report of the Committee of Enquiry into Speech Therapy services. Now there are many courses which the College recognises as leading to a qualification to practice. They will all have different biases and characters depending upon the institutions in which they are housed and the disposition, talents and philosophies of the people who created them. In particular there will be varying amounts of emphasis on the contributions of medicine, linguistics, education and psychology. All must be represented though if the course is to gain official recognition, for communication problems call upon the qualities of doctor, linguist, teacher and psychologist. Any individual who combined all these separate qualifications would be a paragon indeed but would be a very, very long time in the making. As it is not feasible to create such giants, nor yet to require patients to make their own choice or amalgam from the offerings of each profession, we need the profession of speech therapy. If it is to retain its identity and the professional integrity which can alone command respect, it must cherish, within the complex academic material which feeds it, a surety of touch in the practical clinical field. It must also be able to command these clinical skills so that they may be placed at the service of any group or any individual with a disorder of communication, however mild or however profound.

The expansion of speech therapy services into new areas of need and interest is notable. A retrospective study of speech therapy suggests that it was first called upon to contribute to those cases whose difficulties in utterance were extremely conspicuous. The first remedial service to be established by local authorities for both children and adults was for stammerers, where speech re-education was seen as the outstanding need. There followed treatment facilities for speech handicapped school children in whom the inability to articulate consonants interfered with intelligibility. It has been a logical progress for the profession to look beneath the articulatory surface to the inadequate processes that have failed to produce it. Indeed speech problems have been referred to as 'the tip of the iceberg' (Griffiths, 1972). The unknown area beneath this tip threatens education, social and emotional skills. Treating the speech symptom is no longer deemed useful unless this contributes to general language support and command.

It has been an equally logical step to try to amend factors predisposing children to speech problems once their connection with the ensuing disorder had been adequately demonstrated. When it was shown that the main linguistic rules were learnt in the first three years of life the effect of language deprivation at that age could be estimated. Consequently much attention has been given to strengthening the mother's part in stimulating the language of her child. This can be seen in those with hearing impairment where parent guidance and parental language training starts as soon as the loss is discovered in infancy. It is shown in attempts to set up language-geared nursery programmes for the socially deprived and also for the mentally retarded who will need increased stimulation and teaching throughout childhood if they are to acquire useful language function. The trend may be seen very strongly also among speech therapists working with cases of delayed speech who keep careful records of the child's small linguistic increments to assess whether he is gaining mastery of the process and if not how and when he should be helped. The speech therapist's own skills have evolved with the trend, putting a premium upon observation and the ability to teach others the significance of linguistic behaviour.

Another direction in which speech therapy has moved is that of non-verbal communication. The logic of this is not always grasped by those who still equate speech therapy with speech correction. However, it is perfectly reasonable in a profession whose prime concern is communication and which therefore must take responsibility to devise alternatives if speech is not possible or is not immediately possible. In treating profound cases of aphasia and anarthria it has become useful to see whether visual or gestural representations can be employed instead of spoken ones. Many of the training foci are the same: attention must be trained; imitation must be inculcated; communicative interaction must be developed; sequential skills must be taught. As the therapist becomes more proficient in working in this area she may be able to extend the work to other abnormal populations such as the profoundly mentally retarded or the psychotic.

This application of clinical skills from the situation in which they are learned to another in which they are novel demands at least three kinds of recognition. The first is the recognition of the essential premises on which the skill was based; the second is the points at which the new situation touches on the old; the third is the way in which it differs from the old. Unless these are carefully considered the speech therapist will find herself unable to justify the time she is spending and unable to assess the progress of the patient. She needs a new set of guidelines but they will be based on the premises she has always used to monitor progress.

The tendency to tackle more handicapped populations is, as has been pointed out, the consequence and also the means of professional growth, but it is hard on students to be expected to recapitulate the evolution of the profession in their own training. Teachers should guard against the temptation to dangle the esoteric before those whose need is to be taught how to master the primary steps. Student training includes all the areas of knowledge that the profession considers necessary to nourish its growth. However it must ensure that the student is equipped to do her first job, that of recognising and changing abnormal speech in those people for whom it is the major or the only handicap. Once equipped with this training and with some small confidence in her ability to use it she may later make her own moves into new territory. So the work of the student starts with the more obvious speech symptoms, misarticulations; word finding difficulties; voice loss; stammering; then, when the connections between cause, effect and remedy have been well worked out transfer may be made to those areas where judgement takes over from precept.

There will come a time in every clinician's work when she will be asked to see a person whose speech problem is completely unfamiliar to her. For the newly qualified this situation is the rule rather than the exception. It has already been pointed out that the experience clinician is guided by clinical memory but the newly qualified who lack this should not despair. E.M. Forster wrote that 'everything is like something, what is this thing like?' Once you have been trained to analyse one communication problem it should be possible to approach another, as the following example shows.

Mrs B is a speech therapist working with young children who have failed to develop normal speech in spite of apparently adequate potential. The children she sees have acquired speech but not the normal or conventional utterance expected for their ages which are between four and seven. She starts by taking the history in the manner already indicated and by interacting with the child and obtaining a characteristic sample of his speech, which she then subjects to phonological and linguistic analysis. She carries out an examination of the child's oral behaviour and associated motor functions and may end up with information which she reports in the following way.

Case report: At the age of 3.3/12 William was able to carry out a performance test of hearing with no difficulty. This showed him to have normal acuity. He appeared to have no difficulty in comprehension and this was supported by his score of 4.8/12 on the Reynell Verbal Comprehension Scale. On the same scale his Expressive Language score was 2.7/12 and was noted by the psychologist as being 'unintelligible without the guidance of the context situation. The score is based upon full vocal plus context-of-situation guidance interpretations'.

Other psychological findings were that 'performance scores show evidence of above average non-verbal functioning and it is possible that his future non-verbal levels will fall into the superior range'.

William was highly animated and somewhat hyperactive during the investigations but co-operated fully and cheerfully in all aspects of linguistic assessment. He communicated by sentences which were frequently telegrammatic and showed evidence of simplification. Systemic simplification was strongly apparent in William's phonology which was dominated by consonant harmony or assimilation, e.g. [bɪgə goʊ] bigger doll
['tʌpɪn laɪ də tʌʔtɪ] something like the country.

William was able to imitate all the consonant vowel combinations expected for his chronological age and this confirmed the hypothesis that the disorder is a linguistic one rather than one associated with impaired motor skills.

William's parents referred to a recent increase in vocabulary and said that he seemed to be using longer sentences. This, coupled with his obvious intelligence and responsiveness suggests that he may be moving into the period dominated by the desire to convey ideas through spoken language. There is therefore some risk that syntax will outpace phonology to the extent that William will become increasingly unintelligible. Speech therapy should therefore be instigated to teach the main phonological features which have not been normally acquired. Emphasis should be placed on auditory discrimination, sound matching and differentiation.

This report highlights many of the skills previously listed, e.g. attention training; listening; auditory discrimination and judgement; imitation; sound production. The therapist is obviously experienced in this area and makes her pronouncements with assurance.

Mrs B is now asked to see a child of the same age who is not yet starting to speak. She presents as a child with severe delay in all aspects of development. Chromosomal investigation reveals 'abnormality with partial trisomy of chromosome 9. The effect of this on the child's development is not fully understood. We are following her progress and would appreciate a report on your findings and any suggestions you can make as to her management.'

The therapist's examination must obviously be carried out at a much lower developmental level than in the previous case with emphasis on pre-linguistic activity. But the targets of examination are still communicative behaviour, oral and motor functions and full case history must be taken, geared towards pre-speech development. Once more the therapist presents her report, marshalling her information in the following way.

Case report: Mary did not use speech to communicate except by single words; 'no', 'me', with very simple consonant/vowel structure. She made use of the consonant 'b' and attempted several words starting with that sound but the words were poorly differentiated and truncated. Vowel sounds lacked definition and speech attempt was generally primitive. When stimulated to imitate babble chains Mary produced a clearer, livelier tone and was able to incorporate 'l' as well as nasals and plosives. At a higher level however she has not established a phonological or sound system and does not appear to have laid down the kinaesthetic patterns which are necessary for speech. In order to produce a variety of speech sounds it is necessary to work in a strongly stimulating manner with a high degree of concentration on the therapist's part in order to keep the child going. The combination of stimulation at a developmentally low level and a strong degree of control is difficult to maintain.

Mary showed some ability to imitate but could not perform a sequence of movements. She seems to be hovering on the edge of representational play and when this break-through comes it may help her to appreciate language concepts and pave the way for verbal language. At present the limits imposed by delayed cognitive development and specific difficulties with representational skills and sequential learning are holding her back in language development.

The difficulty in acquiring spoken language is compounded by poor muscular control of the speech organs associated with impaired motor co-ordination overall. This adds up to a formidable handicap in acquiring spoken language and also in acquiring a non-verbal system of communication which relies upon representational and sequential skills. Mary needs help through a number of specific approaches to particular difficulties rather than by attempting to find one underlying factor.

Through discussion with Mary's parents we agreed that they should concentrate on helping her representational play and thereby also her concentration and sequencing ability. Speech therapy should start at once with measures to promote direct imitation of movements leading to imitation of speech movements and babbling. Time should be spent at this level in laying down the motor and auditory patterns for speech. Both parents and therapist will work to develop Mary's interest in sounds and speech and help her to listen to simple statements. It is to be hoped that increased maturation will bring these major activities together so that words can be taught. When this is achieved a programme of systematic language building may be instituted.

The areas highlighted are those that have already been indicated but the level at which they are tackled is much lower. While the therapist cannot be expected to have experience of many such children she is able to transfer her knowledge to the area of discussion and make some suggestions that may prove helpful. In both cases it is incumbent upon her to keep a careful record of changes that do take place so that the usefulness of her recommendations can be checked. Thus she continues to build up her own knowledge and render herself of increasing value to the community she serves.

3

The nature of the procedures

It will be apparent from the preceding chapters that the speech therapist works on a basis of information collected and by means of questions posed and answered and observations made. The two basic, broad questions to be answered are: 'what is the kind of difficulty this person has?' and 'what kind of person has this difficulty?'.

The first of these questions is being answered more effectively now than it was before because we have access to much more information than did our predecessors. This information includes knowledge yielded from the results of tests properly selected and applied and from the results and suggestions of colleagues in allied fields. The second question is probably no better answered now than it has been for many years in spite of the increased ways of assessing personality. It is doubtful whether such procedures, interesting though they are, have improved markedly on the clinical insights offered by those speech therapists able to enter into the feelings of the people they are trying to help.

For the last 30 years speech therapy has been practised by people showing a high degree of sensitive insight and capacity for thoughtful character evaluation. The influence of psychologists and psychiatrists has always kept the speech therapy profession in touch with the complexities of human behaviour. In addition, and most importantly, those who were drawn to the work were people with a deep and practical interest in how people behaved and communicated. Frequently this attraction had been initiated by personal knowledge of friend or relative handicapped by speech difficulty. As there was little in the way of status or financial recompense to entice people into speech therapy its adherents were people with a strong sense of service and devotion to their fellow human beings. The attraction of unchartered territory drew people with enthusiasm and initiative. Present day students are therefore well advised to study the individual case histories and therapeutic directives published by those comparatively few pioneer therapists who did venture into print and to lose no opportunity for discussion with clinicians experienced in the work.

The present day speech therapist is required to give a clearer account for herself than was the case with her predecessors. It is no longer enough to know that certain methods are helpful. We need to know why they have proved so and in which circumstances they may prove helpful again. Students are being taught critically to evaluate treatment claims and to try to separate the methods used from the person using them in order to predict whether the methods are likely to be successful elsewhere.

It is highly important for the development of treatment that the right questions are asked in the first place and correct inferences and assumptions made. If this is done treatment will be successful, the procedures justified and the diagnosis confirmed. If treatment is unsuccessful, the assumptions underlying it must be carefully checked and probably changed. These alternatives are illustrated by the following cases of delayed speech in two young boys.

Child A: Referred for investigation of hearing and speech and first seen at the age of 3 years 8 months.

Case history:
Revealed no departures from normal development except a delay in the use of words at around 2 years and subsequent slow speech development. Behaviour was excessively apprehensive and immature. Speech assessment revealed immature phonology and syntax: voice quality was hypo-nasal and there was intermittent mouth breathing. The child 'responded more confidently and with increased speed to raised tones of voice. He did not appear to hear soft speech nor to understand fully statements made in conversational tones which were complex or lengthy.'

Assumption: Speech delay due to hearing loss.

Audiological testing: Revealed losses by air conduction of 40-45 decibels across the speech frequencies in the right ear and 45 decibels in the left. Bone conduction levels were 5-10 decibels across all frequencies.
Impedance measures showed very poor pressure compliance with negative middle ear pressures of minus 250mm of water.
Speech discrimination levels as tested by the Kendal Toy Test were 50/55 decibels.
'this is a clear indication that a significant hearing loss is present.'

Assumption: Supported.

Management: Otological opinion sought and condition investigated and treated by adenoidectomy and myringotomy. Language stimulation and training programme instituted through parent guidance. Focus of training:

Listening
Auditory discrimination
Vocabulary
Sentence expansion.

Audiological re-assessment after 2 months showed normal hearing in both ears through the range 250 Hz to 4 kHz.

Speech re-assessment after 5 months showed well formed sentences and comprehension slightly in advance of C.A. when tested by the Reynell Developmental Language Scale. Phonological system showed 'resolving immaturities.'

Conclusion: Diagnosis correct; treatment appropriate and successful.

Child B: Referred for investigation of hearing and speech and first seen at the age of 3 years 3 months.

Case history:
Stated that all developmental milestones had been passed at the normal time except speech which had been delayed from inception. Behaviour showed frequent temper tantrums and was generally immature with hyper-activity. Speech assessment revealed immaturity in all aspects of verbal expression and comprehension problems allied to difficulty in maintaining attention.

Assumption: Speech delay consequent upon auditory dysfunction.

Audiological testing: Revealed variable responses but mainly within the range 55/60 decibels. It was not possible to carry out impedance testing but the nature of the other findings suggested a likely conductive component to the hearing loss.

Management: Otological opinion sought and examination confirmed presence of fluid. Condition treated by adenoidectomy and myringotomy.

Assumption: Supported. Language stimulation and training programme instituted through parent guidance.

Audiological re-assessment after 4 months showed variable responses within range 50/55 decibels. Echolalia was noted.

Assumption: Questioned. Language re-assessed and psychological investigation carried out. This revealed scatter of results in both verbal and non-verbal tests. Expressive speech level was thought to be around 18 months. Non-verbal items ranged from 23 months to 41 months.

Management: Language training programme re-directed and carried out by the therapist. Focus of training:

Attention
Auditory discrimination
Vocabulary building
Auditory sequential training
Syntax development...
Sentence expansion.

Audiological re-assessment at 4 years revealed normal hearing. Speech assessment at 4 years 2 months revealed continuing difficulty in maintaining attention to speech; echolalia; immaturity in all aspects of verbal expression; simplified phonological system. Original assumption no longer considered adequate to account for symptoms. It was not compatible with the continuing attentional difficulties which kept performance around the 2 year level.

Conclusion: Diagnosis not correct or not sufficiently comprehensive.

Management: Now concentrated on attention control; auditory discrimination; comprehension training.

These two children show some superficial points of resemblance but one case is much more complicated than the other. In such cases there is always a danger, not altogether avoided here, of picking on one outstanding feature without giving enough attention to others less prominent. Failure to observe all aspects of the child's behaviour and to look for an explanation that covers them all can lead to a lack of balanced appraisal of causal factors. Children who present with delayed speech frequently show a picture of contributory factors influencing each other in a complicated and subtle way rather than any one cause. This merits the setting up of a series of sub-goals in therapy rather than directing everything towards the one target.

This can be seen in a third case, another 3 year old boy presenting with speech delay.

Child C: Referred for investigation of hearing and speech and first seen at the age of 3 years 9 months.

Case history:
Showed delay in all developmental milestones. These were noted by his father, the referring physician, who also drew attention to a squint for which the boy was receiving treatment. There had been

several episodes of otitis media. Behaviour was mature, independent, amiable and co-operative.

Speech assessment: Showed severe expressive retardation but good comprehension. The child vocalized with a variety of inflections to convey meaning. One or at the most two-word combinations were attempted consisting of simple consonant/vowel utterances using nasal and simple front plosives. Vowels were poorly differentiated. No back plosives could be produced in imitation.

Assumption: 'it seems most likely that he is suffering from developmental delay in motor and perceptual skills with speech as the most highly synchronised and complex skill being most affected. It is likely that verbal language is being further depressed by hearing loss associated with past episodes of otitis media.'

Audiological testing: Revealed air conduction levels at 50 decibels across the speech frequencies with normal bone conduction. Impedance curves were very flat with poor compliance and negative pressure on both sides.

Management: Otological opinion sought and condition treated by tonsil and adenoidectomy and myringotomy. Speech therapy instituted on a weekly basis to combine specific language work and parent guidance. Focus of training on:

Imitation
Sound production
Discrimination
Modelling and
Sentence expansion.

Audiological re-assessment 3 months later showed normal levels with speech discrimination at minimal.

Further investigations included psychological evaluation which showed non-verbal intelligence to be within the good average range. Verbal comprehension as assessed by Sheridan and Reynell scales was 4.6 to a chronological age of 4.1.

Re-appraisal after these examinations led to amendments in management. Test evidence suggested that the good verbal comprehension and intelligence would promote development of syntax. The parents were advised to concentrate on language input by reading and talking to their son and also to expand his utterances as demonstrated by the speech therapist. The latter would concentrate on the production of sounds and words to help the child expand his phonological system and experiment with word use.

Progress excellent and steady. Assumptions supported and management directives confirmed. In this case no specific diagnosis was made but all relevant factors were properly considered. Treatment developed from the profile of strengths and weaknesses derived from observation and testing. The appropriateness of the management was proved by the child's rapid, steady and sustained improvement.

In the first case, that of Child A, the developmental history was clearly given by the parents who had two older sons with whom to compare this one. They believed him to be having much more difficulty in understanding and acquiring speech than the others and were concerned about possible hearing loss. The child's immature and shy behaviour raised questions as to immaturity being strongly associated with speech delay together with his position in the family. It was possible that he was being over-protected and had learned to manipulate his family by his immature speech and behaviour.

It is wise before exploring such questions too deeply to see whether such a child's behaviour can easily be accounted for by the major assumption of cause. In the case of conductive hearing loss the fluctuating levels can cause confusion in young children with a consequent withdrawal from speech situations. Discrimination of speech is likely to be reduced and the child thereby lacks confidence in his own speech as well as the words of others.

If the child is particularly sensitive by nature he will be more penalised in his relationships with other people and thus in his emotional development than will the more robust and independent child who will pursue his individual course without necessarily feeling too concerned by the effect of other people's apparent vagaries. Thus the personality of Child C did not appear to be adversely affected by the loss but the more diffident nature of Child A was affected. The possible effect of the loss on Child B is difficult to assess but it is likely that it increased his difficulties in attention considerably by adding a further confusing element. His withdrawal was probably exacerbated though not caused by the hearing loss. However, whereas in this child the loss could not easily account for the behaviour, it could in Child A. Relief of Child A's hearing loss was therefore the first target rather than further assessment. The correctness of the procedure was in fact confirmed by the child's progress without any other management being required than speech and hearing guidance. Progress was measurable by hearing and linguistic re-assessments. The linguistic management of the child through parent guidance also proved helpful and did not increase the child's dependence on his mother. Rather it increased confidence on both sides thus dispelling any idea of neurotic dependency.

In the case of Child B the initial case history was not full enough to justify the assumption that was made concerning the importance of hearing in relation to other factors. Parents do not always give a full picture on their first appearance at a clinic. They are sometimes unsure of what is required and frequently overawed or ill at ease. Not infrequently there is a very natural desire to present everyone in the best light which leads to suppression of unpleasant facts. There is also inexperience in assessing the significance of behaviour of a first child, as was the case here. It was difficult for this boy's parents to know whether the child's lack of ability to relate to them and attend to their speech was normal for his age or not.

With this child we have the combination of withheld information on the one hand and too broad an assumption on the other. Fortunately the picture started to be filled in fairly rapidly as management progressed. The whole course of treatment, guidance and educational placement was a long one, with periodic re-assessment and guidance from the psychologist and regular language training from the speech therapist replacing audiological counselling. In addition to general buttressing or support, both workers had to adopt crisis intervention tactics when particular stresses appeared. This dual role of anchor man and trouble shooter must be accepted by any therapist working with handicapped people.

The third boy, Child C must also be considered in the round. It was interesting that his parents, both medical people, had not suspected hearing loss because they saw the slow development of speech as perfectly compatible with growth in other areas. The boy's natural independence and ability to occupy himself meant that he was not constantly drawing their attention to any inadequacies.Parents tend not to be worried about happy purposeful children who are gaining in accomplishments even if slowly, particularly when the slow rate is something the parents understand and for which they are prepared. It is in cases like this that an outside observer can be most useful and it was indeed the nursery teacher who first drew attention to the pronounced speech delay and suggested further investigation. Although her suspicions were justified and treatment was certainly needed the parents were essentially correct in their fundamental belief in their child's ability and potential. This was shown by the progress which he made. Had the intervention been delayed for much longer however the picture might have been different.

These histories show the assumptions that therapists make and the procedures they carry out in individual cases. If several cases with similar features are seen a hypothesis may be made about the nature of the condition. For example conductive hearing loss was not formerly thought to affect the acquisition of speech and language unless it was severe. Even then it had nothing like the effect imposed by perceptive or neurosensory loss. As the result of more regular and sustained acquaintance with such children, some therapists started to question the relationship between fluctuating hearing loss of a conductive type and acquisition of the morphological features of language. The hypothesis was that as so much information about language forms is carried by unstressed syllables, e.g. 'ed' and consonants of low acoustic strength, e.g. 's' or 'z', the child with a loss of varying severity might have difficulty in the mastery of these forms. Such a hypothesis needs to be tested experimentally before it can become influencial in clinical practice but it typifies the way in which professional growth takes place.

Another example of hypothesis testing may be seen in the case of children with chromosomal abnormalities. The author had occasion to analyse the speech of two XXYY children and was impressed by the resemblances in utterance and behaviour. Discussion revealed that similar and more extensive observations had been made by Garvey and the same conclusions drawn. The hypothesis tendered was that children of this type were unable to lay down the kinaesthetic patterns for articulation and thus failed to develop a phonological system. This hypothesis will need support from further and more extensive studies but it is a good illustration of the pursuit of something interesting and potentially significant (Garvey and Kellett, 1975).

A much more extensive hypothesis was tendered by Morley in relation to articulatory disorders in children. At the time of investigation many such conditions were grouped together under the classification of dyslalia. This broad grouping failed to designate the subjects of particular interest to Morley. She identified a subgroup consisting of children who were unable to improve their speech production by attention to auditory discrimination or other aspects of language learning and who required active assistance in imitating and producing sounds. The designation 'articulatory apraxia' was made on the assumption that there had been a failure of neuromuscular learning during the stage of speech acquisition. Treatment then focused upon imitation training and conscious control of articulatory movements. The success of the treatment methods supported the hypothesis and these methods have now passed into general clinical use. The medical aspect of the hypothesis, that the responsible lesion lay somewhere between that giving rise to spastic dysarthria and to motor aphasia, has since been subjected to continual examination.

Greene (1963) in summing up much of her earlier work, hypothesised the existence of two main groups within the broad classification of language delay. The first was composed of children whose problems consisted mainly of motor programming. The second group showed perceptual, discriminatory and general language learning problems. This interesting hypothesis stimulated further investigations and was helpful to those ideas currently being pursued independently. The group of motorically handicapped children bore some affinity to Morley's group but more to that subsequently described by Edwards (1973) under the heading verbal dyspraxia. The language learning group has proved interesting territory for psychologists attempting to predict or ameliorate educational failure. It has also been the target of much investigation by linguists trying to establish the breakdown of systemic phonological and syntactic features.

Hypotheses concerning the nature of language breakdown may be tendered by several different professions, each of which proceeds to make its checks in its own way. Neurologists now have access to the CAT scanner in supporting or negating hypotheses as to the localisation of language function and the relationship between language behaviour and sites of lesions. This is the first time diagnosticians have been able to note the actual position and size of a lesion at the same time as carrying out assessment of function. The availability of the CAT scanner has consequently given very considerable impetus to the work of research groups trying to account for the changes that take place in language as the result of pathology and then during the process of recovery.

It will remain much less easy to assess the effect of small lesions on the nervous systems in developing children. Detailed longitudinal studies must be kept and such studies well correlated before we can have much confidence in asserting the exact effect of neurological dysfunction on the minutiae of language learning. All professions interested in this area are likely to develop closer checks on the effect of one impaired function on the acquisition of a related skill rather than looking for a neuropathological substratum to every case, even though it is strongly suspected.

Short term auditory memory failure has been postulated for some years as an important feature in developmental language disorder. The speech therapist may be alerted to the possibility through the child's speech behaviour; the presence of open syllable; reduced temporal span; impaired prosody through failure of rhythmic and verbal sequencing and reduced phonetic patterning with consequent phonological constraints.

The psychologist will be alerted by educational problems and by inconsistences in the learning profile. He may place particular importance on certain sub-test findings in the WISC and ITPA in testing out his assumption. Both professions will be interested in looking at the child's long-term auditory memory as a source of possible compensation in remedial activities and will also have an academic interest in the possible relationship of the two types of memory which could engender further hypotheses.

The speech therapist has always depended upon other professions to check her therapeutic hypotheses but there is some professional movement now toward taking over this responsibility, particularly in language breakdown. This has come about through the new attitudes of enquiry and healthy doubt already described and because the profession now has more assessment tools of its own to enable checks and comparisons to be made. A brief review of three cases of acquired dysphasia treated by the author at intervals of 11 years may be of interest here. In each case the speech therapist was reassured by the progress of the patient that some useful therapy was taking place but very much needed tangible and documentary evidence that this was so. Such evidence is necessary for any therapist to keep her honest and to quieten her clamorous therapeutic conscience which always suggests that something further could be done. It is also highly important for the patient to have some objective check on his ability and progress, a point well made by Butfield (1958) in writing of her notable collaboration with Zangwill in the field of aphasia rehabilitation. The following summaries show how the cases were managed.

Case history: Mr A. first seen in 1957, aged 56–referred for speech therapy some 6 months after c.v.a. suffered abroad. Initial assessment made only by speech therapist and based on work by Butfield (1946) and Eisenson (1954). Subsequently referred for general rehabilitation and assisted by occupational therapy.

Evidence yielded from assessment and therapeutic trial suggested predominantly expressive dysphasia. Language therapy was carried out entirely by the speech therapist and devoted to language building in all areas using speech, reading, writing, dictation put into practical effect through a variety of techniques. After 2 years of twice weekly speech therapy the patient was then taken to see a linguistic phonetician for advice in developing techniques of word finding and self monitoring (Trim, 1967; Byers Brown, 1971).

Case history: Mr B. first seen in 1967, aged 49–referred for speech therapy immediately following admission to hospital after suffering c.v.a. whilst on holiday. Subsequently transferred to the author on return home. Assessed on Minnesota Test for Differential Diagnosis of Aphasia 10 weeks after c.v.a. and re-assessed on the same test at intervals during the following 12 months. Full audiological and psychological evaluation carried out at the end of the first year following c.v.a. Patient given a battery of tests for dysphasia, educational attainment, intelligence and verbal reasoning. Programme of language re-education subsequently worked out between speech therapist and psychologist (Byers Brown and Ives, 1969).

Subsequent therapy carried out by the speech therapist alone. Seen in 1975 by linguist with whom he followed a subsequent programme of systematic psycho-linguistic exploration (Cruse, 1978).

With these two patients the entire onus was on the language rehabilitation. While linguistic and psychological assistance requested by the speech therapist did yield valuable academic and research stimulus it was not approached entirely with that aim. Assistance was sought by the speech therapist to ensure that everything possible was being done to help the patient regain his language.

Case history: Mr C. first seen in 1978, aged 59–referred to the author 2 months after c.v.a. for investigation, with the consent of the speech therapist who had been working with him since onset of aphasia.

Full assessment carried out using Boston Diagnostic Aphasia examination. Profile drawn up and therapeutic programme instituted. At the same time results of the Minnesota Test were compiled by the first therapist together with therapeutic implications. Both sets of findings were discussed by the two therapists and common areas agreed. At different stages of therapy jointly carried out, findings were checked against both diagnostic profiles and progress noted.

Once more the emphasis is on rehabilitation but there is another trend. Here we see speech therapists using the means at their own disposal to check that their treatment is well designed and relevant and that it yields results. For this they are not applying to members of other professions but to their own. It seems likely that this will be the path we will take in the future. While we will continue to work in the closest co-operation with other professions we will also attempt to satisfy ourselves by comparative assessments and evaluations that our therapy is effective. We are no longer so dependent upon other professions, e.g. medicine and psychology to do this monitoring for us.

In areas where very precise delineation of a cause is not only important but actually available, speech therapy is very properly subservient to other professions in establishing this cause. An example is the elucidation of hearing loss, particularly its nature and degree in young children. Another is the exploration of palato-pharyngeal activity by new mechanical aids. The speech therapist has three main duties here. The first is to make the right observations initially so that the patients may be properly referred and investigated. The second is to learn how to interpret the scientific and technological information yielded by these investigations and the third is to assess how well the results explain the nature of the speech disorder. It is not likely though that therapy can be checked against improvement in hearing or palatal growth. The check provided against faulty diagnosis is in these cases of a different order from those provided against faulty therapy. Speech therapy leads to improvement in function and this is something still only partially amenable to scientific proof. As has been shown, speech therapists feel their responsibility to measure that what they are doing does actually help the patient to improve in the manner purported and this is very important. The academic satisfaction of the therapist must always be secondary to the welfare of the patient. Therapy exists to explore any avenue that offers genuine promise of improving the patient's well being. Morley, in a classic text, reminds us that 'although some of our time must be occupied with the clarification of thought and growth of knowledge, as therapists we are concerned primarily with the *patient* who has the disorder and not only with the disorder itself.' Any hypothesis tested and any exercise practised is still done with this aim in view.

4

The process of problem solving

Once the existence of a problem has been recognised and its nature established the process of problem solving can begin. The process will continue until the best possible adjustment has been achieved between the speech handicapped person and the demands placed upon him. If the speech therapist has to abandon her treatment before a satisfactory level of attainment and adjustment has been made she must do everything she can to see that access to future speech therapy is not closed to the patient should it be later deemed appropriate. She should also attempt to provide support from other agencies in the interim period. The speech therapist's responsibility to her patient throughout the whole period of his need has been indicated in Chapter 1. The therapeutic process or the business of problem solving will involve many areas of activity. An essential aspect is being able to gauge where the pressures are likely to come from and when. Therapy demands sustained endeavour on both sides. There will inevitably be times when this endeavour flags and when there is discouragement. The patient and his family may be disappointed at the slowness of the progress or discouraged because after a promising start there is a plateau period where everything is happening beneath the surface. Many promising ventures have been abandoned because they did not yield the speed of change that characterised the original impetus.

The speech therapist must be able to control her own reactions so that she is able to judge properly. She should also learn early how to work with colleagues and other allies. Working with a regular clinical case load involves the complicated aspect of human relations and the different but possibly equally complicated matter of practical arrangements. A beautifully prepared treatment cannot be carried out in the absence of the patient. It is necessary therefore not only to devise a suitable therapeutic programme but to ensure that it is offered at a time when the patient can attend. If he is unable to attend because of transport difficulty or parental apathy the therapist must see that means and escorts are provided. The combination of practical arrangements and emotional burden can weigh heavy upon the young clinician who will not have realised all that was being done by others during her period of student training. The student is therefore well advised to participate as fully as she can in all the aspects of her training. This way she will share the duties of her supervising clinician and not allow herself to be cushioned from the impact of different but coinciding demands. The cases touched upon in earlier chapters will now be used to show how treatment proceeds. Cited on page 12 was the case of a child of 2 years 8 months who presented with arrested language development following an encephalitic type illness. The investigating team was listed. We will consider the period when the speech therapist was predominantly responsible for the child's management. This followed his referral by the pediatrician and lasted until he was placed in a language unit — a period of more than 2 years.

Emotional background to the problem

Both the child and his parents have sustained severe emotional shock. The child has suffered pain, fear, distress and frustration. The parents have suffered agonizing anxiety during the acute phase of the child's illness and are now in a state where joy at his physical recovery is intermixed with fear as to the extent of any residual handicap. They need the re-assurance of being shown the child's strengths and healthy attributes, one of which will be the normal auditory acuity which has been demonstrated. The therapist will then emphasise the importance of this skill in the re-learning of speech and for linguistic and educational growth. The child needs the re-assurance of pleasant, stable, relaxed handling and of having his communicative efforts understood. Granted the needs on all sides, an early step must be to find a place where the child may best receive regular help. Where best can he be assisted to experiment in language and be trained in its associated skills?

Therapeutic environment

The child may at first appear to best advantage in his own home. His surroundings will be familiar and he will be free from any apprehension associated with hospital or medical treatment. A home visit will therefore be invaluable in showing how the child behaves in normal circumstances and the conditions in which his parents are trying to cope with him. When this initial visit has been made the place of regular treatment must be determined. There are three main choices:

1. The child's home

2. The play group or nursery
3. The speech therapy clinic.

The child's home is not likely to be suitable as a permanent site for therapy. The child will want to play and otherwise behave as he normally does and the presence of his familiar toys will rapidly pass from being a welcome comfort in the therapist's eyes to being a most unwelcome counter-attraction.

The child's mother is also likely to be distracted towards the usual domestic tasks or small crises with which any home is assailed. As a result neither child nor parent will then be able to co-operate in a programme of attention training leading to language development. Moreover the familiarity of the background may prevent the parent from seeing the child's behaviour objectively.

The nursery school or the play group may appeal because of its apparent potential for language stimulation and its real stimulus towards play, but it could be the worst choice for a child who has attentional difficulties and impaired comprehension. He will be over stimulated and the atmosphere of excitement and competition which can easily be built up among small children will be bad for him. He will lack the inhibition to prevent himself being caught up in the activities of his peers.

Neither of the above alternatives should be eliminated automatically however. If the home has sufficient space and no other small children are clamouring for attention there could be a place found for regular work. If the nursery also possesses withdrawing and private places and has a high ratio of staff to pupils it may be suitable. Wherever the child is treated he needs a quiet room with reduced visual stimulation and the minimum of claims competing for his fleeting attention. The particular strengths and weaknesses of both home and nursery must be weighed against those of the speech clinic. There the therapist and child should certainly hope to find quiet and pleasant surroundings. However, in spite of much effort to raise the standard of speech therapy accommodation in community clinics, this is not always so. This child must be treated in a community rather than a hospital clinic so that a new chain of pleasant links may be forged. A medical atmosphere should be avoided as, indeed, it should for most children. If the clinic is suitably quiet and pleasant it is the best place for the child's therapy. At least one parent must be there throughout treatment and visual and other distractions must be kept to a minimum. The therapy session must be free from interruption by person or by telephone. A tape recorder must always be available because the child's developing utterances are of prime importance to the therapist.

After he has gone she must be able to make notes on his behaviour, listen to his recorded speech and analyse his utterances. If these conditions cannot be complied with the therapy session is not maximally valuable to the child and will not be a guide to his potential and prognosis.

Forward planning

The speech therapist must be able to look ahead and to prepare the parents and those who have responsibility for educational provision for special school placement. If the preparation turns out to be unnecessary nothing much will be lost, but if the therapist has not made adequate preparation the child's progress may be severely disrupted and his parents will experience shock and helplessness rather than understanding and acceptance. It is not helpful though to keep dwelling on the future unless something is happening in the present that will increase the parents' faith in her judgement and allow her to make a realistic appraisal of rate of language growth. In addition to creating a therapeutic environment the therapist must use it for the application of treatment techniques. She must also continue to seek out information in the following areas:

1. Brain growth, specialisation and shift of dominance
2. Conceptual development and cognitive growth
3. Linguistic development.

Careful record keeping is essential not only to assess this child's progress but also to contribute to the progress of future children through research. Every novel patient is a research subject. Information on such cases should be shared with the other speech therapists and offered in suitable form to colleagues in other professions. The speech therapist will also seek guidance from colleagues in trying to fill in the blank areas in her own understanding.

Such information can be exchanged during the case conferences which are a regular feature of good clinical practice, or the exchange may take place in a special conference or workshop designed to concentrate the attention of several professions on a particular problem area (Byers Brown and Beveridge, 1979).

A major difficulty in working with a child of this kind is our lack of knowledge as to how one aspect of language and behaviour affects another. Broadly speaking we know that in language development comprehension precedes expression or recognition precedes production and that language systems are built up one step at a time. Whereas a normal child moves fairly smoothly and swiftly from one stage to another, a handicapped child such as this one may experience plateaux. During these resting periods it is hard for the therapist to know how much to demand and how much to feed in. This doubt in her own mind means, of course, that it is extremely difficult for her to guide other people. In a case such as this the therapist must experiment with language stimulation techniques, keeping a careful account of what she is doing. Improvement will come about through a suitable method given in a suitable manner at a suitable time and in a suitable place.

Management

The therapist must make clear to the child's parents what she is doing and what she hopes to achieve both explicitly and by example. The example is given by the way she speaks to the child and the demands she makes on his understanding. It will be shown in the kind of play she encourages him to develop. She must make it clear to the child's mother that the relationship she is offering the child is not an absolute model for the mother, who has her own and much more important relationship with him, but there will certainly be aspects of the clinical relationship which the therapist can with advantage share with the mother. Almost certainly there will be a tendency among the whole family to over protect the child and to indulge him. The therapist may be able to help by setting limits and allowing the mother to see what controls are helpful and why. Explicitly the therapist may seek the parents' help in language building. She will show them the appropriate length of sentence to use and to encourage. She will show them classes of words which the child may find easy to master and those he will find difficult and give as clearly as she can the reasons for this classification. She will be able to anticipate or at least explain subsequently why the child showed regressive behaviour when he became excited or confused. These discussions will help to lessen the parents' anxiety by increasing their understanding and by giving them practical ways to help their child. It will thus prepare them for any special recommendations which will have to be made because they will understand how these conclusions have been arrived at. In return the parents will feel the obligation to share with the therapist their views on the child's progress and their concern and plans for his future.

The problem in this case was that of the child's condition. It did not lie in his personality nor in the attitude of his parents. There will be very many cases in which the problem lies almost entirely in one or the other of these two. While the speech therapist will make every effort to worry out the problem for herself she will very likely want to enlist the help of colleagues. In the case of personality difficulty her major ally is likely to be the psychologist. In the case of entrenched attitudes of apathy or hostility on the part of the parents, the ally may be the child's teacher, the general practitioner, or the health visitor. Practical means to ensure the child's attendance will be the first order and then painstaking work to gain the parents' interest and trust. It is not naive to think first of practical matters. Attendances at speech clinics will be precluded as often by expensive and fatiguing journeys as they will by lack of interest or hostility, but if these attitudes exist they must be tackled. If the therapist is deemed the best person to do this she will show as clearly as she can the possible consequences of the continuing handicap and not hesitate to give strongly worded warnings as well as offers of help. Such admonishments are part of the therapeutic process. No child can learn a new skill unless the ground is prepared for its use.

The two children cited in Chapter 2 as attending Mrs B's clinic have different problems necessitating different approaches. In both cases fortunately there are no immediate difficulties in co-operation and support, but the stresses are there and must be catered for. The small boy was described as having a very restricted phonological system. This, combined with his active interest in communication, his rapidly developing syntax and semantic growth meant that he was becoming less rather than more intelligible with age.

Emotional background

The parents will first be worried that there is something actually wrong with the child's speech apparatus. They must be re-assured on this point. His normal auditory acuity and good intelligence must be emphasised as the assets they are. The problem of his lack of intelligibility must then be discussed. It is very distressing for parents not to be able to understand their children's speech. The mother particularly feels that she is constantly failing her child when she should be, of all people, the one who can act as his interpreter.

Therapeutic background

In this case, regular treatment sessions at the speech clinic are almost certainly the best way of working.

Management

The onus is fairly and squarely on the therapist to come up with a technique helpful to this child. She will first carry out a thorough phonological analysis and find out what rules are present in his system. She will then have recourse to the literature of language acquisition to work out what the therapeutic steps should be. She will be guided by the need to improve intelligibility as soon as possible without cutting across developmental areas to the extent that the child cannot take the next move for himself. She must find for the parents, some way of helping their child so that he becomes more intelligible to them. This will mean restricting the child's statements during his period of speech practice so that he has opportunity every day for normal, conventional speech which can be understood by others.

Work with the parents of a child like this will be very specific. It will show them the steps towards change. It will enlist their aid in effecting this change. To give a simple example; the therapist has shown the child the difference between the labial nasal continuant [m] and the labial voiced plosive [b]. She provides plenty of material to help him enjoy producing and identifying the sounds and contrasting them with one another. She will then want to generalise the concepts of nasality and plosion. The child's family may help considerably by giving him plenty of practice at the different stages.

1. Key words taught by therapist:
   'Hum' and 'Mummy'. Re-inforced at home in the form of a game.
   Child 'hum, Mummy'. Mummy complies.
   Child 'No more humming Mummy'. Mummy stops. Variations on the commands can be given as long as the sounds are limited to nasals and vowels.
2. Key words taught by therapist.
   'Bye-bye' and 'Bobby'. Re-inforced in action.
   'Bye-bye' is said whenever possible. If there is not a useful 'Bobby' in the family a toy so named must be provided.
3. The therapist moves on to teach words combining the phonemes and emphasising their structure:
   'Number one' etc
   'My number'; 'Mummy'(s) number'
   'Bobby'(s) number'
   'No more number (s)'.

Re-inforcement at home could be given with a toy telephone, a specially constructed bingo-type game or whatever appeals.

The therapist then moves on to generalising the contrast between plosive and nasal and so uses other placements. Key words may include 'under' 'bingo' 'hungry' 'dinner' 'Ben' (a brother for Bobby) and thus; 'no more dinner Ben'; 'where'(s) Bobby'(s) dinner?'; 'under the table'.

At this point voice and voiceless forms may be brought in to contrast with those already mastered.

Any statement of actual happenings will always appear ingenuous, but we have to work at many levels at once. Appreciation of rules of language is not in itself helpful to parents in improving intelligibility. They are likely to want to do something definite and practical. It is for the therapist to appreciate the rules, undertake a proper analysis and then give the parents very clear suggestions for fun and games for the family. The parents and other children will be able to understand what the child is saying and he will have the pleasure of knowing this.

The stresses borne by those responsible for the management of Mrs B's second case are of a different order. This little girl will inevitably be enrolled for many years in a programme of diagnostic therapy. As she shows ability to benefit from this programme or as she does not, she will reveal other signs or symptoms which will demand investigation. For the physician in charge of the case and for the speech therapist carrying the burden of communication, there will be dual concerns which could appear to conflict. The one is to follow up every lead which could give more information as to the child's state. The other is to keep the family unit from being destroyed by the constant search for an answer and to help the parents to enjoy their daughter without continually seeing her in pathological terms.

Emotional background

This will be one of anxiety about a condition not fully understood by anyone. Everything that is known must therefore be shared with the parents. While it seems cruel and unhelpful to keep examining a child solely to underline her deficiencies, it is helpful and positive to explore every way of helping her at every stage of her growth. Full investigation should be seen by everyone as a means of ensuring that the best decisions are made at the time when they have to be made.

Therapeutic environment

Whatever the arrangements of the speech therapy service in the area, this kind of child should always be known to the member of staff who is likely to be permanent. In the structure of services as it now exists, the newly qualified therapist will work in a team, responsible to her Chief Speech Therapist who is ultimately responsible to the Area Speech Therapist. In practical terms such a child as this will probably fall to the Senior Speech Therapist who is building up a speciality in work with the structurally impaired or educationally sub-normal child. The child's parents must feel that if this therapist should move on or leave for other reasons there will be someone in the area that knows what has been done and what must be tried. There can be few experiences more disheartening than to have one's handicapped child constantly being appraised and discussed by those who do not know of her state, her growth and her individual ways. The problem in this kind of case is of prediction and it will be exacerbated by lack of continuity in management.

Management

This may have to include investigations as to the structure and competence of the oral mechanism, which could require attendance at highly specialised centres for oro-facial malformations. Genetic and pediatric/neurological investigations together with psychological assessment will also be required. Case conferences will therefore involve many disciplines. While a medical practitioner may be the best person to co-ordinate all the relevant information it could fall to the lot of the speech therapist. Even if it does not do so officially she is likely to find that the mother will use her as a safety valve and a confidant and thus she may receive invaluable information and insights which she must share to the advantage of the child. At the same time she must be able to offer a number of alternatives in the way of communication. If the child responds to representational training leading to simple spoken language, this must be fully developed. If the spoken avenue is not accessible a non-verbal communication system can be offered while investigations into lingual and palato-pharyngeal competence are being carried out.

Finally we should consider the problems presented by the adults to whom brief reference has been made. The case of Mrs A. cited in Chapter 1 shows a problem arising from a mixture of emotional and adaptive factors. Such cases are not unusual and have been well described notably by Greene (1972). The solving of this problem is likely to need a combination of specific vocal re-training and general support.

Emotional background

This is likely to be one of anxiety. The otolaryngologist will have attempted to dispel fears as to the presence of malignant disease but they may linger. If so they will interfere with progress as well as general well being. It is important therefore that a practical change in voice quality is effected as soon as possible. The person may very well be one who feels unduly concerned to carry other peoples' burdens or alternatively to live her own life to the full. The motivation behind her behaviour must gradually be uncovered by the patient and the therapist during their work together. The therapist may wish to employ some kind of personality inventory in addition to her case history and vocal analysis.

Therapeutic environment

The best place for this patient's treatment would be a room of good size and pleasant aspect without medical connections and without childish accoutrements. If the patient is seen for therapy in the hospital speech clinic together with laryngectomised and other surgically and medically dependent patients it will be very difficult to assure her that she has no medical problems. The atmosphere should encourage easy conversation and reinforce the link with normal activities. The room should also be big enough to allow Mrs A. to carry out exercises in vocal projection, including singing, without inhibition or interruption. If a suitable room is not found there will be no real opportunity to build up the patient's voice and so once more treatment will be inadequate and prediction uncertain.

Management

As has been indicated, this will be a compound of teaching vocal principles and vocal hygiene and exploring those factors in the patient's personality and relationships which makes it difficult for her to put them into practice. If necessary the patient's husband and other members of the family should be seen and their help enlisted. All circumstances which place particular demands on the voice should be fully explored with the patient. This kind of problem should admit of fairly speedy solution. While the therapist should guard against relapse and should not terminate treatment too precipitately she should not see her role as one of long term mainstay.

With the aphasic patients described in Chapter 3 the long term relationship between therapist and patient must be accepted as a necessary part of the therapeutic management.

Emotional background

These men can no longer see themselves and can no longer function as confident, competent people moving easily among personal and professional communications. They are reduced and diminished in their own eyes and in the eyes of others. Unless the speech therapist can command their trust and confidence nothing that she attempts will be useful. Unless she can find strong allies to help their wives and to give them the essential stimulation and support, she will be unable to raise their level of language function and maintain it. To take on such patients without being able to count on the support of other people places a heavy and continuous burden on the therapist. This can cause her to become tired, to lose her capacity for thinking up interesting and helpful things to do and thus it can lead to resentment of their demands. The speech therapist needs in these cases more than in most to be clear sighted in what she can undertake.

Therapeutic environment
There are four main possibilities for the carrying out of therapy.
1. The person's home
2. The stroke club premises or community centre
3. The speech therapy department of a hospital
4. The rehabilitation centre.
These may all be used at varying stages of therapy. Much will depend on the extent of the associated handicaps. In the cases of these three men none of the possibilities listed can be deemed entirely satisfactory as the sole and regular place of treatment. Such patients must not be imprisoned in their homes for the very disability from which they suffer is imprisoning enough. The community centre might seem the best alternative but it is not conducive to hard work and these patients need to work hard towards their own recovery. The speech therapy department may be suitable but if it is one also used for children it can be demeaning in its aspect.

The rehabilitation centre is the most likely place for the patient to develop confidence in his recovery and it is grievous that so few of these centres are available to the aphasic patient by reason of his communication problem alone. Most are reserved for the physically handicapped person who needs the services of physical and occupational therapists. It may well be up to the speech therapist to adapt the most suitable of the clinics in the area for the care of aphasic patients using a combination of group and individual treatment. This has been done very effectively in Blackfriars under the auspices of the School for the Disorders of Human Communication. If the place of therapy is unattractive, the journey long and tiring, the transport uncertain and the opportunity for conversation minimal the therapist will not succeed in her work however good her techniques and inspiring her manner.

Management

There will be continuous and necessary interchange between techniques of language investigation and re-building, environmental exploration and support. These will be discussed more fully in another chapter. The speech therapist will assess her patient's communicative skills in a way which is helpful to him and his family as well as to herself. She will devise procedures to improve language structure and function which make sense to him and in which he can co-operate fully. She is trying to reconstruct his living language and she cannot do this without his full participation.

The process of problem solving must be seen in all its aspects. Amongst the colleagues on whom the therapist will rely for support will be academic and research orientated people. From them she will learn more about the conditions she is treating. On the other hand her allies will also be those who are close to the patient, as from them she will learn about him as a person. Finally she must call on those who can make the necessary practical arrangements for his treatment and support. Each problem will have its own focus; the communicative disorder, the personality and attitude of the patient; the circumstances which exacerbate or perpetuate his condition. If solutions are to be found there must be flexibility, resource, and above all stamina in their pursuit. When considering the focus of the problem it is highly important to uncover evidence which will suggest what the rate of progress is likely to be. Therapists become very rightly worried when a patient fails to move as fast as was predicted and, as has already been said, they may abandon treatment which might have been successful if properly timed. A useful concept here is the biochemical one of the *rate determining reaction*. For a process to be completed a series of sequential reactions has to occur. One of these will determine the rate or progress of the whole sequence. If the sequence contains the elements A, B, C, D, the process may be represented diagrammatically as follows:

$$A \longrightarrow D \qquad \text{whole sequence}$$
$$A \rightarrow B \rightarrow C \rightarrow D \qquad \text{component parts}$$

The component B may determine the speed and ease with which the following stages are encompassed:

$$A \rightarrow B \rightarrow C \, ? \, D$$
$$\text{Rate determining reaction.}$$

If this reaction fails to occur there will be two effects. The one will be a failure of development to the next stage. The other, associated with it will be a build up or accentuation of activity at the early stage.

We can see this concept applied to the speech clinic if we use the three boys cited in Chapter 3. We are attempting to predict the kind and rate of change in each of these boys once the apparent block to progress – the conductive hearing loss, – has been resolved. In predicting the rate of change in any child we ask ourselves 'what does the child actually possess that is going to enable him to make progress?' The rate determining factor will be the child's ability to make use of what he is given. Each boy has been held up at a certain point by failure of auditory acuity. They are all thus retained at a very early stage of speech acquisition and language growth:

Process

A	B	C	D
hearing $\longrightarrow$	discrimination $\longrightarrow$	auditory sequencing $\longrightarrow$	language units for communication

If this diagram represents the process the next one will show where the boys stand.

A	B	C	D
?	X	X	X

The series of sequential happenings is, for a time, arrested. We then intervene at point A and improve each child's ability. Thus the move to B is possible. If the whole sequence is now to take place the activity around B is crucial. The area B $\rightarrow$ C harbours the rate determining reaction. *Child A*. Evidence shows that this child was able to make full use of his new acuity and that he consistently built upon his hitherto restricted language structures. We may thus hypothesise that the rate determining reaction was one of auditory discrimination and judgement. The child had been prevented in the past from using this properly but once it was available he was able to move steadily on. We may therefore represent his growth thus:

A $\longrightarrow$ B	$\longrightarrow$ C	$\longrightarrow$ D
hearing discrimination	auditory sequencing	language units for communication

The essential reaction at Point B occurs and the rest of the sequence is able to take place.

Child B. This child was not able to make use of his new-found acuity to move on through auditory sequencing to language mastery. If we hypothesise the same rate determining reaction, – that of auditory discrimination – we are left with the following representation.

A ──────► B   X   C   X   D   X
hearing   discrimination

This child is unable to move on because the rate determining reaction, which in this case is auditory processing, is not operating effectively. Thus he stays where he is linguistically but also builds up the factors which are present but which are not able to be extended. He becomes echolalic, using the skills he has, consolidating and reinforcing them but not moving on to the normal linguistic development.

Child C. In this case we see again the release of the apparently blocking agent at point B but we have a different result.

A ──────────► B ──────► C ──────────► D

In this case the linguistic process is not just encouraged but accelerated by the emergence of element B.

This child was able to capitalise on his new found acuity to move into the learning area in which he was competent. His performance here was a good predictor of his essential linguistic competence and this was manifest in the speed and completeness of his language mastery.

If we refer back to the diagram on page 11 in which the language model is presented we may hypothesise that the rate determining reaction in these children operated between *auditory acuity* and *auditory processing* and this determined the development of *comprehension, symbolic formulation, conscious analysis of sounds* and *internal language*. These subsequently found expression through the intact motor pathways leading to *spoken language*.

In the case of the little girl, Mary, seen in Mrs B's clinic the rate determining reaction lies at a different point. The therapist's report makes it clear that progress in this child will depend upon her ability to move on to a higher conceptual level. Once she is able to use an action or a sound to represent something else the various subskills which have been taught may be combined to give her language. The length of time it takes her to move to this level will determine the kind of language structure and use which she will ultimately achieve. The importance of this aspect was therefore very properly spelled out by the therapist.

If we look at Mary's position against our language model we can see that her arrest is at the following level:

Auditory processing↔*Memory*↔*Motor activation and processing*

above that there is as yet no movement so the whole sequence which will result in *spoken* or *non-verbal language* is held back. If it is held back for a long period, it may never be entirely set in motion or satisfactorily completed.

With many patients *memory* is the rate determining reaction. On our model we can see it intervening to facilitate comprehension; to make use of imitation and to link auditory and visual representations with motor performance. If the child or adult is not able to retain a verbal pattern accurately enough to reproduce it he cannot be expected to add to his word store or language matrix at a rate sufficient to generate *speech*.

If he is very slow to improve in retaining syllables and words, the whole process of language growth or language recovery will be predictably slow and probably limited.

Mentally retarded children and adults will have considerable difficulty in making use of information that they are given unless the ground is carefully prepared and the information supported. Granted the generally slow rate of language growth in the mentally retarded, the rate determining reaction in an individual may well be triggered by the early language stimulation he receives. Very young normal infants may learn sounds or words as items (Cruttenden, 1979) and only subsequently go on to learn the rules which govern their use in a communication system. Mentally retarded children may not move on to rule learning until a much later stage and then may learn the rules incompletely. If at a young age the child is given increased language support and teaching he may do better. Much work among the mentally retarded is devoted towards this end (Jeffree and McConkey, 1976). Therapists working with mentally retarded persons in adult training centres have found that 'item learning' is still a conspicuous characteristic and that linguistic rules which allow for the generalising of one taught pattern are not available. This missing attribute slows and restricts all linguistic growth (McCartney and Byers Brown, 1980). It may be hypothesised therefore that failure to grasp the significance of rules at the normal time is a feature of limited mental capacity but that failure to learn it later is associated with lack of teaching. Once a person starts responding to and using a limited number of cues only it is extremely difficult for him to make use of others. The rate determining reaction is the response to rule teaching. If the opportunity is not created, the reaction cannot take place.

A rate determining reaction is certainly not confined to physical or intellectual features. Embargoes upon learning arise as often from anxiety or despair. A distressed child is in no condition to respond to teaching and neither is a depressed adult. Failure to learn pseudo voice after laryngectomy may be because the patient rejects the whole concept of himself as a maimed individual. The whole business of the operation with its uncomfortable and messy sequelae and the reduction of personal identity is so traumatising that the patient has no wish and no energy to create a new persona and a new method of communication. The rate determining reaction here will be his ability to come to terms with his condition. If it is not functioning his present state of despair and helplessness will be built up correspondingly.

Another determinant will be the relationship between the therapist and her patient. If at her initial interview the therapist can create confidence and optimism this will engender energy and thus allow activity to take place. Frequently she is lucky in that the patient's personality and hers are in accord. If this is not the case she is, of course, the one who must make the initial effort to accommodate. If the early stages of the relationship do not go well the rate of progress is likely to be slow. There are many therapists who have distinct preferences for certain conditions and they are rightly encouraged to specialise. While all speech therapists are trained to a level of overall competence there should always be opportunity for individual specialisation. The treatment of stammering is perhaps the clearest example of a condition where the interest and enthusiasm of the therapist is the determining factor in the success of therapy.

The rate determining reaction of the stammerer is likely to be the extent to which he is able to tolerate behaviour which he has previously refused to accept. Thus the adult stammerer who comes for treatment with strong motivation to change and who retains that feeling is going to make progress. Should his motivation flag he will be buoyed up by the energy of his clinician until he has re-captured it. If his motivation and tolerance are low his rate of progress will be slow and if the therapist's confidence in her methods is also low this progress will peter out altogether. If his initial move into fluency is blocked his stammering reactions will be intensified.

The speech therapist cannot be expected to solve all the problems that come her way. Even when she receives the maximum of help from colleagues and from the patient's family the problem may defy solution. She will continue to work best and be happiest though if she feels that she has sought for a solution in a sensible manner and considered all the influencing factors. If the problem cannot be solved she may then wind up her therapy without self-flagellation. A frequent instance where the cards are stacked against her is when she is dealing with a child who needs more help from home or school than either is willing to provide. The speech therapist sees the child for a very limited time. If both of his major environments are adverse her efforts, however considerable will make little difference. Given this situation the conscientious therapist may often feel that she must persist in order that the child receives some support, but she should also consider the effect on her employing authority when it is noted that the child has attended for four years and is still unintelligible.

Speech therapy holds a peculiar position in that it places highly developed skills before people but with very little authority to demand that those skills are utilised and supported. The therapist has the responsibility for stating the nature of the problem and laying out the contributory factors. She must then determine the proper approach and try to ensure that the focus of her therapy is directed towards the area where it will be most effective. She will do her best to see that the practical circumstances in which treatment is given assist that treatment. In exchange for this care she has a right to expect a fair measure of recognition and co-operation. If these are not conceded the problem is likely to remain unsolved and the therapist must accept this with as much equanimity as she can muster. Happily the experience gained will almost certainly advantage another person in the future and lead to a higher quality of care for those waiting to respond to it.

5

The nature of the equipment

The past chapters have dealt mainly with the attributes and
behaviour of the clinician herself in seeking to effect a change in
her patients, but these skills and attributes may be considerably
extended by the use of suitable equipment. Attempting to describe
equipment that may be useful to the prospective clinician at the
dawn of the silicon chip era is equivalent to instructing someone as
to how to improve his arrowhead before sending him off to war.
One will be out of date before the print is set. This chapter will not
then seek to itemise equipment that may be found useful in the
next decade, but will rather seek to discuss why equipment is
necessary and how it should be devised. The word equipment is
not only intended to designate elaborate hardware. It can be
applied to the toys, books and small domestic accessories which
serve the therapist well in setting up communicative enterprises
and developing individual skills. Indeed until recently these hum-
ble accessories were the speech therapist's main stock in trade.
Many heads of departments were hard put to explain to the management why boxes of straws, crayons, bags of cotton wool and ice
lollies featured as the major items on their equipment lists.

The making of equipment always appeared on the curriculum of
the speech therapy training school, greeted with more or less
enthusiasm according to talent. It was naturally accepted that a
student should be able to turn her hand to making a puppet and
running up an articulatory 'snakes and ladders'. It was also
accepted that a large bundle of pictures cut from magazines must
be the constant companion of a speech therapist so that they might
be at any moment stuck into the 'speech book' to evoke an errant
consonant or shown to an aphasic patient to stimulate description.
The necessity for creating on the spot equipment persists. It is notable that the report of the Committee of Enquiry (Quirk, 1972) in
suggesting the use of speech therapy aides specifically mentions the
usefulness to the speech therapist of someone who can make and
repair equipment. The ability to draw an immediate portrait of the

child in question or to create an instant breath direction exercise is enviable and a great aid to motivation and rapport. So we are unlikely to see the speech therapist ever totally dependent on scientific and commercial enterprise for her devices. Also we are too small a body to tempt companies into creating many special lines for us alone, but the move towards that end is well underway as a glance at the following record will show. It is not intended to be a comprehensive list of available equipment, but simply a representative one.

The purposes for which the equipment is necessary have not changed but the number and complexity of the items shows a very considerable growth during the arbitrary 30 year span chosen. Here are some of the items available to the speech therapist and her colleagues:

Purpose of Equipment	1950	1980
To give information on the structure and function of the organs of speech and hearing	Pure tone audiometer Soft tissue X-ray Image intensifier Cinematography	Pure tone and impedance audiometers. Apparatus for recording evoked responses; electrocochleography; electronystagmography; vestibular function recording; electro-palatography; video-fluoroscopy; nasendoscopy; nasal anemometry CAT scan; fibro-optics
To record performance	Recording apparatus (disc) Phonetic transcriptions Unstandardised tests of articulation and language Standardised tests of intelligence, vocabulary and educational attainment Film	Tape recorders, reel to reel and cassette Phonological and syntactic analysis Film, television and video-cassette Standardised tests as previously and also for aphasia and all aspects of child language Stammering severity inventories.
To give the patient more information about his performance	As above Mirror	As above Voiscope; real time speech analyser Repeat-recorder Language master Biometer Palatal training devices

Purpose of Equipment	1950	1980
To stimulate the patient to make a change	As above	As above DAF Edinburgh masker Relaxometer
To allow patient to compensate for inadequacy	Hearing aid Prosthesis Vibrator	As above; also devices used previously but now produced in a variety of forms and made of light, flexible and durable materials
To provide alternative means of expression to speech	Signing Writing	Paget Gorman system Blissymbolics Makaton Amerind Splink Possum
To maintain interest in treatment	Progress records Toys Games	A great variety of specially devised games and programmes

The outstanding point to be made from this comparison is that we are seeing a strong move towards the use of electronic apparatus not only as a diagnostic tool but as a treatment aid. The cost of such items as voiscopes and speech analysers will determine their regular use. With the development of silicon chip technology they are going to be available shortly at a price we can afford and in a size that makes them practicable for even the peripatetic therapist to use. Those of us whose first introduction to recording came with the disc cutting machine have no difficulty in comtemplating the development. In a major London teaching hospital in the 1950s the recording apparatus was housed in a separate cubical as indeed it needed to be for it consisted of three large items, each of which could only be lifted by two strong and determined people. With apparatus of this kind there is little chance of quickly capturing a significant speech signal thrown up during a routine treatment. Neither was it possible to record a patient unless he could come to the apparatus. Information on the very early stages of speech recovery which could be taking place in the ward was not available. The difficulties that arose when trying to capture the speech of very young children will be obvious and they prevented the attempt being made by all but the most resolutely research minded.

Now the use of the cassette recorder is so widespread and its quality so good that no therapist can be excused a thorough and meticulous attention to the speech of her patients. It is possible to capture the random utterances which may be so illuminating not just in content but in structure. It is also possible to retain the record until linguistic analysis has been carried out. We have seen developments in the use of tape recorders comparable to those in electronic calculators. When these were first introduced they were no better than a good slide rule and very much more expensive. The increased accuracy they yielded did not, for most people, compensate for their cost. Now a pocket calculator costs no more than a good slide rule; it is more accurate and it can do far more. So it has become the natural companion of all who have to carry out even the simplest calculations as a regular feature of their occupation. A further analogy can be made with the hearing aids now produced for children and revolutionised by the transistor and miniature battery. We shall certainly see corresponding developments in the visual display systems or training devices.

The development of a piece of apparatus will give considerable impetus to treatment techniques and may radically change the techniques offered. Past language and speech work with the severely deaf tended to be analytic and to require specific attention to individual language items. While this could produce articulate speech in the intellectually gifted it could not engender speech that was easy for the ordinary listener to understand. Nor could it offer the variety of linguistic forms that are used in normal conversation. The speech directed by the teacher to the pupil was slower than normal and exaggerated in pronunciation, so that although the pupil might grasp the word meaning and therefore make sense of the message, he was only receiving very limited messages and these in special form.

With the advanced technology to produce high quality amplification in a form tolerable even to a young child, the techniques of language teaching altered radically. Young children whose handicap had been identified early were given amplification and their parents involved in guidance programmes with all the emphasis on natural speech. Parents were shown how to speak to their children, not by using limited and unnatural input but by using a rich and redundant language so that the child could pick up a variety of constructions and concepts. This exposure to natural speech developed in the child the essential prosodic features of speech which contribute so much to intelligibility. With further developments in visual display systems the older children will be shown how to monitor their pitch and stress so that a more natural sounding, less conspicuous utterance can emerge. Speech teaching for the deaf is now carried out at the speed and with the rhythm of normal utterance. We see here equipment at its best; an extension of the talents of the teacher and therapist. It enables her to use her own speech in a way that will help the handicapped child to learn not only 'the trick of language' (Fry, 1979) but many attributes of its performance.

If the therapist elects to use equipment additional to her own ears, tongue, eyes, wits and hands she will do so for the reasons already stated, namely:

1. To give her further information about the nature of the mechanism and to establish as exactly as possible the structure and function of the relevant organs
2. To record as many aspects of the patient's performance as she can and in the most convenient way
3. To give the patient more information about what he is doing and thereby enable him to start making his own deductions and accommodations towards improvement
4. To stimulate him not only towards these accommodations but, if necessary, to make a radical change in the manner in which he receives or expresses language
5. To allow him to compensate for a physical handicap, a structural defect or a traumatic injury by the use of a prosthesis or other piece of apparatus designed expressly for the purpose
6. To combine and develop both the last two activities by teaching a whole new language system as an alternative to speech
7. To maintain interest in improving his performance through what may have to be a very prolonged remedial process and one where the rewards are not immediate

If the therapist decides to purchase special equipment she will obviously be biased towards those items which will be of use to a large number of her patients. This kind of equipment is also likely to be the most reasonably priced since it will have a good market throughout the speech therapy service. Those items which remain expensive are the ones individually tailored for one person. There are in fact many considerations which affect the purchase of equipment and the student should be exposed to these during her training so that she does not approach them naively when she sets up her own clinic.

Considerations

1. A piece of equipment may be sought if the therapist will not be able to get the required information by any other convenient method

2. The most valuable first piece of equipment will be one absolutely basic to the discipline within which she is working
3. If a highly specialised piece of equipment is contemplated it
must be relevant to the area where expertise is required
4. Before making any expensive purchase it is necessary to ask
whether the existing clinical equipment is adequate and if not
whether this piece will be a major improvement. Will it do
something a great deal better than anything that is in the clinician's possession already? Will it enable her to do something
that she cannot yet do or that she cannot yet do very well?

The same questions can of course be asked about inexpensive
equipment also but here correct decisions are not so vital. Five
pounds worth of inappropriate card games will not set back further
development very notably, but 500 pounds worth of unused electronic appliances in the clinic cupboard is bad for the clinical purse
and for the clinical reputation.

BASIC EQUIPMENT

The outstanding piece of equipment in the speech clinic is the tape
recorder and it is difficult to see how any competent therapist can
now function without one. Just as with the purchase of a car the
family will extend itself in all sorts of ways and change the whole
organisation and rhythm of its life, so has the tape recorder determined the direction of clinical growth. Speech is transient. A
statement is essayed and completed before the listener has had time
to focus his attention. The speaker may be asked to repeat but few
people are capable of making even the briefest statement several
times in exactly the same way. If the speaker is a small child the
chances of exact repetition are very remote indeed. Therapists who
have to rely upon phonetic transcription for their only records are
therefore forced to work with very small speech samples at a time.
Thus we have the long established use of the stimulus picture and
the one word response. To rely upon this for remedial purposes is
the equivalent of testing the child's walking ability by taking a
series of static pictures.

The tape recorder has enabled speech therapists to avail themselves of the techniques of linguistic analysis which have been the
major transformers of our clinical approach. From the linguists we
have learnt how children acquire language with a degree of detail
which gives us the ability to predict as well as describe. We can
now analyse speech on the run with all its variability and character.
To use the techniques of phonological and syntactic analysis, we

must be able to listen to the same spoken passages over and over again. We could not do this without the tape recorder. While this may be its major contribution to our professional growth there are many other ways in which it is immediately and permanently helpful.

People need to listen to themselves very objectively if they are to make any changes in the manner of their production. It is almost impossible to do this while speaking or to recall the exact quality of an utterance once spoken. Playing back to the stammerer, the dysarthric or the dysphonic the message which has just left his mouth will convince him as will no amount of comment and description. The manner in which such treatment sessions should be handled will be discussed subsequently since preparation is obviously needed for listening objectively to one's own speech. Without labouring the point further then we can simply summarise the contribution of the tape recorder as highly notable because:

1. It allows flowing speech to be captured and replayed for purposes of analysis
2. It enables the patient to listen to his own speech in order to note its features and attempt to change them
3. It enables the child or adult to listen to his own speech against the model of the therapist's and thus be able to make use of the latter to effect the change
4. It allows an exact record to be made of the changes taking place in the speech of the patient
5. It allows the therapist to listen to herself talking in a variety of clinical circumstances and thus allows her to work out the possible effect of her words and manner on the people concerned
6. It allows clinical interviews to take place and histories to be recorded without the interruptions occasioned by note taking and thus allows the dynamic relationship between the people concerned to develop naturally.

The tape recorder thus qualifies as a piece of equipment basic to the core discipline in which the speech therapist is engaged and it will be interesting to see how it is superceded in the future. The present generation of students will take as naturally to video-recording as to audio-recording and this has some marked advantages. The non-verbal accompaniments to the spoken message which contain so much information can also be captured. The pre-speech skills of the small child can be recorded and analysed as can the behaviour of the speechless adult. We are offered through video-recording a further dimension to the processes of taking in and analysing the information which we have learned to do auditorily. We are also given the situational cue which is frequently essential in worrying out an unintelligible utterance.

Further developments in equipment making are likely to build on the ways in which human behaviour can be swiftly and easily recorded and reproduced and these can only aid clinical practice.

SPECIALIST EQUIPMENT

Purchase of specialist equipment is necessarily related to the task for which it is intended and the centre where it is to be housed. In any one speech therapy service there may be a special assessment centre where complicated diagnostic procedures will be carried out. These procedures will need a team of people and so the centre is expensive by virtue of staff time as well as equipment. At the moment there is considerable disparity of access to specialised centres for investigation and treatment. Recommendations have been made in Government reports as to the number and siting of specialist diagnostic units and centres of excellence. Several kinds of institutions can be envisaged in relation to speech therapy. Firstly there is the centre developed and renowned for a particular kind of expertise. Examples would include:

The Royal National Throat, Nose and Ear Hospital and the Nuffield Centre

The Wolfson Centre of the University of London

The Phonetics Department of the same University at University College

The Blackfriars Centre for Dysphasic Adults at the School for the Study of Disorders of Human Communication

The Camden Re-habilitation Centre

The Cheyne Centre for Spastic Children

The Department of Audiology and Education of the Deaf of the University of Manchester

The Hester Adrian Research Centre of the same University

The Department of Speech and Voice Pathology, Victoria Infirmary, Glasgow

The Plastic Surgery Unit, Canniesburn Hospital, Glasgow

The Stroke Research Unit of the Frenchay Hospital, Bristol

The Department of Linguistics Science, University of Reading.

This list is of course an exemplar merely and not a directory. Each centre offers a particular kind of expertise and will draw to it patients who are thought to need this care. The centre will then generate, in addition to specific patient reports, more generally applicable research findings and treatment directives. We need a number of specialist centres and that number has not yet been decided. Each region should have access to one for advice on communication disorders but some of them will remain nationally rather than regionally active. They may be expected to have a team of highly qualified staff and equipment which is so expensive to purchase and maintain that it can only be justified if used nationally. In exchange for this privilege the centre may also function as a teaching unit enabling others to benefit by its findings and ensuring that these findings are properly interpreted.

The number and siting of centres for developmental assessments is at present under consideration following the receipt of the Committee of Enquiry into Child Health Services (Court, 1976) and into Special Educational Needs (Warnock, 1978). These centres would be expected to house experts in all areas of child development with the appropriate tools of their own trade and also ones for this particular job. They may also be expected to feed much information back to the local services thus obviating the need for expensive and time wasting duplication.

In addition to those centres which house colleagues from different disciplines sharing equipment and procedures, any speech therapy service will attempt to establish a central clinic which will house its more expensive, specialised equipment. All therapists may have access to this and the expense of purchase and maintenance may be justified by the number of patients served. The range of equipment collected there will depend on several things. The first is the amount of money the local authority has to spend and is prepared to spend. A second is the availability of similar equipment near at hand. The third and very potent factor is the eloquence and determination of the Area Speech Therapist or deputy in demonstrating the need. If a rural area is being served the service may benefit best from a mobile clinic containing essential and robust equipment which can be transported to any isolated site. If the service is based on a large urban population it may justify a wide range of special equipment housed in the clinic most easily accessible. This can then be the site of intensive and even residential courses where the equipment is used to maximum benefit in treating a large number of patients and also in training students.

The student must therefore be exposed to methods requiring a high degree of technical expertise even if she is not immediately able to make use of them in her clinical practice. Unless she has seen the procedures she will not be able to make the appropriate referrals nor study the ensuing technological developments. While it will be the responsibility of senior staff to recommend and purchase they usually welcome the advice of juniors fresh from training in university, college and polytechnic departments where equipment is tested and demonstrated and where teams of people are available to discuss its merits.

It would not be appropriate to deal with equipment for speech therapy entirely in terms of major purchases. The materials housed in the community clinic will certainly see as much use and therefore need as much thought. We may consider the selection and use of equipment and materials in relation to the language model used in Chapter 1. The numbers on the diagram show the points of breakdown and the forms of remediation (Fig. 2).

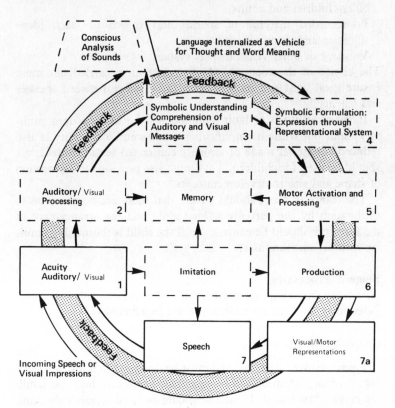

Fig. 2 Language model showing focus for training

Stage 1: Acuity

If auditory acuity is at fault it will be necessary to carry out full audiological investigation. The child or adult will be referred to a central clinic where suitable personnel will be able to administer tests for acuity, discrimination, balance, pressure and localisation as indicated by the audiological responses. The patient may then be referred back for help with language training, speech production or voice monitoring.

Speech therapy equipment

Forms to present and collate phonological and syntactical analysis

Language trainer or other amplification as prescribed by the audiologist

Toys to encourage representative play in young children

Picture cards and books to encourage sequential narrative in older children and adults

Pre-recorded material of sounds and speech to teach identification and discrimination

Voiscope or other visual display system.

The choice of the room in which treatment is carried out must ensure good light and room to vary the distance between speaker and listener.

If visual acuity is at fault attention will be focused upon auditory input but without amplification (unless auditory acuity is also reduced). Material made of strongly contrasted texture substances should be used for children. Toys must also provide for exploration of shape and size to develop concepts.

The choice of room should ensure that there are no obstacles to exploration by the partially sighted child and the arrangement of the furniture should be constant until the child is thoroughly familiar with his surroundings.

Stage 2: Processing

Assistance in estimating the degree and nature of the processing defect may be given by audiologist and psychologist.

Congenital cases (auditory)

Young children: The material must be designed to improve listening. Auditory attention can be encouraged by sound toys and familiar noises. Pre-recorded material should be used to teach discrimination. Visual material, objects, pictures and sequencing cards should be used first then transfer made to the auditory modality. A language trainer set low may be used to encourage auditory concentration. Some apparatus, e.g. portable pure tone audiometer should be used to train responses to sound signals of varying length, pitch and volume. This may also be used as background noise to build up discrimination and selection of foreground-background sound. Language master and loop recording of simple statements with accompanying pictures may be used for comprehension training.

Older children: Material on the same lines but with emphasis on word discrimination; pictures and objects of similar phonemic construction or semantic association to teach discrimination and judgement. Good quality recording machine for the child to use on his own with pre-programmed material. Cartoons to be studied accompanied by pre-recorded explanation or narrative.

Acquired condition in adults
Assessment material to include standardized tests for aphasia. Teaching material as above but with suitably mature material. A variety of reading material will be needed.

With both children and adults visual displays may be used if they do not confuse. They should be essayed with caution. The choice of the room should be made predominantly on the grounds of quietness and lack of strong visual distraction.

Speech therapy equipment (to include the following material)
Developmental movement charts
Material for sensory stimulation and proprioceptive facilitation e.g. ice, brush.
Tests for astereognosis
Palatal training devices
Electro-palatogramme
Biometer
Relaxometer
Visual display system
Mirror.

Stage 3: Symbolic recognition and comprehension
Assistance will be gained from the psychologist.

Stage 4: Symbolic formulation and expression

Speech therapy equipment will include:
Large and small objects for representational play
Drawing materials

Young child
Large and small objects for representational play

Drawing materials

Objects for categorising by shape, colour, size and kind

Dolls house, toy village, wooden cut-outs to be assembled in representation of domestic happenings.

Older children

Photographs and pictures representing familiar activities

Apparatus for model making

Drawing material

Language programme or teaching scheme e.g. the colour pattern scheme (Lea, 1970)

Video-tapes showing simple sequences of activity accompanied by narrative then without so that child may supply her own.

Variety of reading material.

Acquired condition in adults

Assessment material to include:

Standardised tests for differential diagnosis of aphasia and allied conditions

Photographs and pictures representing familiar activities

Video-tapes showing simple sequences of activity with and then without accompanying narrative

Reading material

Young children with disorders of this kind should be treated in language units where group work can be employed. Older children should be taught in special schools or units by teacher-therapists or by both teachers and therapists working together. Adult aphasic patients need the accommodation described in Chapter 4.

Stage 5: Motor activation and processing

Assistance will be gained from physiotherapists.

Stage 6: Production

Material as above together with the following *speech therapy equipment*:

Voiscope

Vibrator

Masker

D.A.F.

Articulatory tests

Dysarthria assessment material

Nasal anenometer.

Stage 7: Speech
Material as previously indicated, together with the following speech
therapy equipment:
  Recording apparatus
  Assessment forms for phonological linguistic analysis
  Vocal and fluency rating scales.

Stage 7(a): Visual/motor representations
  Paget Gorman
  Blissymbolics
  Makaton
  Amerind
  Splink
  Possum
  Writing materials.
Many of the patients requiring equipment outlined above will be
physically handicapped. They may therefore appropriately receive
treatment at a school or centre for the cerebral palsied or a rehabili-
tation centre. Those with structural abnormalities of the oro-facial
mechanism or who have suffered laryngeal surgery may be most
appropriately treated in a specialised centre in the first instance.

It is not yet possible to expand on equipment which will assist in
the coupling of the auditory and motor systems and markedly
improve the feedback circuits. This is, indeed, the major problem
in assisting patients who have severe difficulty in regulating speech
output in the absence of hearing loss or paralysis. We await further
research into neurophysiological function before we can expect
many developments in the control of monitoring. The speech
therapist is still therefore highly dependent upon sensory stimulation and direct imitation to improve performance whether in children or adults.

Experiments with programmed learning to date suggest that
although remedial programmes can be administered by other people (instructors at training centres, volunteers, speech therapy aides
or helpers) the skill of the professional therapist must be involved
at all stages of the programme's construction and in the analysis of
data.

We may examine a recent project of this kind (McCartney, 1979
and McCartney and Byers Brown, 1980) to see how the equipment
devised can bridge the gap between the special skills of the professional speech therapist and the social, educative and supportive
aims of a group of instructors.

The experiment was carried out in an adult training centre to devise audio-visual programmes of language training for the use of the staff. Such a centre exists to train severely sub-normal adults in practical and social skills which will enable them to contribute to and be accepted by society. A key factor in society's acceptance will be the ease with which the handicapped person can make himself understood. If a trainee is not intelligible or if his manner of speaking makes him conspicuous and causes embarrassment, the staff of the centre will be very properly concerned. Research carried out into the needs of the adult training centre staff (Whelan and Speake, 1977) showed a strong desire for more access to speech therapy which reflected that concern.

We therefore have on the one hand a large group of adult severely sub-normal persons deemed to require speech therapy and on the other a small body of professionals. It is highly unlikely that any area health authority will be able to afford a speech therapy service which will provide individual therapy for each member of the severely sub-normal population who requires it. So the following picture emerges:

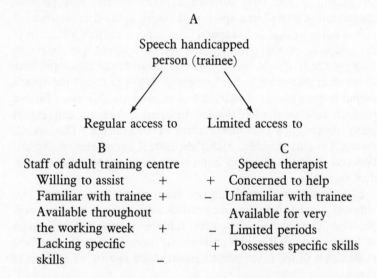

A

Speech handicapped
person (trainee)

Regular access to   Limited access to

B   C
Staff of adult training centre   Speech therapist
  Willing to assist   +   +   Concerned to help
  Familiar with trainee +   −   Unfamiliar with trainee
  Available throughout   Available for very
  the working week   +   −   Limited periods
  Lacking specific   +   Possesses specific skills
  skills   −

In order to convert all the − signs or debits to + or credits we need to select those specific skills which C can offer and graft them on to B. As C has taken a long time to become trained in her area of professional expertise such an operation is unlikely. An alternative would be to devise a programme in which the professional knowledge of C could be systematically set down to subserve a number of tasks which B could administer. A final refinement would be the construction of a piece of apparatus by C which would embody those tasks so that B could concentrate on his chosen role of teaching and support without the onus of keeping all his activities canalised into the one programme.

The speech therapist and instructor need to carry out a task analysis with the therapist giving the lead. It may be decided that A's speech is rendered less than easily intelligible because of the absence of the sound 's'. The speech therapist analyses the trainee's speech to find out whether the sound is represented in his system. Analysis reveals occasional use of 's' in medial and final positions.

1. Analysis fails to reveal use of 's' to signal plurality, but reveals some approximation to 's' in initial positions; never in clusters.

Programme focus – auditory discrimination; auditory memory; rule learning.

2. Analysis fails to reveal instances of normal production of 's', but reveals some attempt to signal plurality by length of vowel or emphasis on last syllable.

Programme focus – production; imitation; repetition.

In the experiment cited, programmes were devised for both such cases, namely speech production and auditory discrimination programmes. They were constructed for one phoneme in one syllable only and were designed to provide structured practice for the trainee on that speech sound. Familiar, easily depicted words were selected and illustrated by photographs for the speech production programme. A series of targets was established by which the trainee could work through from the production of the selected sound in isolation to the production of the trained sound in untrained words. This procedure was supported by re-inforcement, modelling, corrective feedback and evaluation of responses carried out by the A.T.C. instructors. Responses were recorded on dual track 'student' and 'master' tapes which allowed comparisons to be made.

Auditory discrimination programmes were presented on a sound slide projector to which headphones were attached. This was linked to a response switch. Taped instructions required the trainee to respond to 'is this a ?' producing a correct word for the illustration or a distractor word. A correct response allowed the tape to advance. An incorrect response stopped the tape.

Trainees were able to work to a routine laid down by the therapist but with support from the instructors. The original representation may therefore be rounded off as follows:

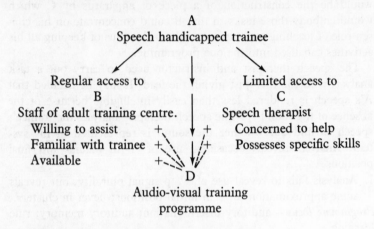

The equipment fulfilled the following purposes:

It gave information about the trainee's performance

It stimulated the trainee to make a change

It maintained the interest in treatment of the trainee and instructors

It allowed all three parties to do something that they could not achieve otherwise.

We can anticipate greatly accelerated development in the construction and use of such programmes. What we cannot anticipate is the extent to which the computer can take over from the human agent in giving suitably fine and selective information to encourage individual endeavour.

6

The nature of the conditions and terms

The scope of speech therapy has now been indicated and there is a fair degree of consensus among speech therapists as to the conditions requiring treatment. Unfortunately this consensus does not extend to the terms that should be used to depict the conditions. The need for a clear and comprehensive terminology is everywhere expressed but not yet satisfied.

A subject develops a terminology when the existing vocabulary proves inadequate for the phenomena it wished to describe. Technical terms allow for the precise and accurate expression of those concepts which would be clumsy and ambiguous if otherwise formulated. A profession, being comprised of people joined together in a common pursuit, needs a language which will give structure and definition to its ideas and enable information to be exchanged succinctly. It may achieve its technical vocabulary by plundering terms from neighbouring professions and incorporating them into its own developing matrix, or it may select this vocabulary more formally by agreement followed up by rigorous enforcement.

At the time when the College of Speech Therapists was founded, some terms for speech disorders were already well established by the medical profession which provided the main model for diagnosis and treatment. These had to be allied with others that the new college wished to propagate and the whole vocabulary related by rational classification. With a teaching and examination syllabus to launch and a journal to publish, the College was very much involved with taxonomy for several years following its creation. It has since returned to that topic many times by creating special committees to review its terminology. The latest is likely to be the most comprehensive in its field of endeavour but is therefore unlikely to come up with any recommendations in a short space of time. So present day clinicians have to continue to cope with terminological difficulties which a greatly expanded syllabus indicates and a very large clinical clientele demands. A strong minded clinician may succeed in maintaining order and conveying meaning by selecting her terms with care, using them consistently, and explaining them when their use could cause confusion, but the student is not in this position. It is not for her to make an arbitrary choice from a number of alternatives without being sure that they will be acceptable. Before pursuing this point however, it may be helpful to see how the present confused position has come about.

The College of Speech Therapists presented in its original classification the four broad areas into which the act of speech could be broken down.

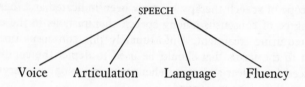

SPEECH

Voice   Articulation   Language   Fluency

Associated with these were equally broad causal categories
Congenital   Acquired
Organic   Functional

Sub-divisions were soon necessary and such terms as Psychogenic, Neurogenic, Habitual, Hysterical and Developmental became incorporated. Under these headings were placed the conditions which were specified by medical terms and then by terms developed by the College. Medical terms made use of Greek roots as the terminology was first propagated at a time when all students received a classical education. Whether the College was justified in assuming this to be the case for its own entrants in 1947 is questionable. It is certainly questionable no longer. To acquaint a present day student with terms of Greek origin is to do little more than to tamper with natural ignorance. The student will learn the terms and use them perfectly well if, as in anatomy, they are rigorously and clearly taught and invariably used for the same phenomena. The student cannot however be expected to show the same command over the Greek terms annexed by speech therapy when each author or clinician invests the words with her own special meaning.

To make the point more firmly: a student could probably fathom out the meaning of the word 'apraxia' and could accept the definition given by the neurologist, but the student would not be able to gather from the mention of that term for a speech disorder whether the speech therapist was referring to 'articulatory apraxia', 'verbal apraxia' or 'lip and tongue apraxia'. Furthermore she would not then know whether the speech therapist considered the term to cover a disorder of imitation, sequencing, timing, skilled volitional movements, a language disorder manifesting itself in verbal production difficulties or a disorder of sensori-motor programming.

Indeed the speech therapy student would not be alone in this ignorance. It will be apparent from the number of associations cited that the word alone will not give the condition specificity. It is just this lack which makes speech therapists wary of using particular terms even to convey information to close colleagues.

There seem to be two choices as to the way out of this difficulty. The first would be an arbitrary and well supported terminology. The second would be to use descriptive terms rather than diagnostic ones. The College of Speech Therapists is at present attempting to use both approaches, as may be seen from its last real statement on the subject in its evidence to the Committee of Enquiry into Speech Therapy services. College evidence included a section headed conditions requiring the care of a speech therapist. This section summarised the postion in the service and in the training schools as to the focus of attention.

CONDITIONS REQUIRING THE CARE OF A SPEECH THERAPIST

1. Delay in the acquisition of speech and language
2. Deviations in utterance with regard to voice, articulation, language and fluency
3. Loss or partial breakdown of voice, speech and language

The College statement proceeded to expand the categories as follows:

Delay in the acquisition of speech and language

Acquisition of speech by the young child is the result of the response of a healthy organism to environmental stimulation. Articulate, fluent speech is the manifestation of language competence. It is associated with:

1. Normal acuity of hearing
2. Normal neurological function regarding the reception, perception and comprehension of sound patterns
3. Normal intellectual development governing the comprehension, organisation and formulation of language symbols
4. Normal parent/child relationship and emotional well-being

Conversely, disorders of communication may arise from:

1. Impaired auditory acuity
2. Cerebral palsy and other manifestations of brain damage

3. Mental retardation
4. Emotional disturbance or immaturity
They may also arise from lack of environmental stimulation or from slow maturation in an otherwise healthy child. Frequently a combination of factors is present.

Deviations of utterance
Deviations from acceptable utterance may be found in the child or adult population as the result of congenital or acquired abnormalities of the organs of speech and hearing; neurological and intellectual impairment; psychological maladjustment or faulty learning. These factors may be present singly or in combination.

Voice disorders
Voice is produced by sound waves originating in the larynx. Vocal abnormalities may arise from structural abnormalities of the larynx. In such cases the speech therapist will undertake vocal training on request of the E.N.T. surgeon in charge of the case. Vocal disorders or dysfunctions are found in those with auditory impairments who cannot adequately monitor their vocal output. They are also found in persons with neurological impairment, notably cerebral palsy, where the activities of the vocal cords are disturbed in themselves or in their co-ordination with other neuromuscular functions necessary for speech. A sub-category of disorders of voice is that of *disorders of resonance*. Here the vocal note is distorted in its passage through the resonating chambers. Causes may be structural anomalies of the upper respiratory tract notably cleft palate. The speech disorder arising from cleft palate affects resonance and articulation. It requires treatment from a team of experts – plastic surgeon, orthodontist, speech therapist – and, because of its frequent association with hearing loss, otolaryngologist and audiologist. The speech therapist is concerned with the assessment of speech prior to and subsequent to surgery and with speech therapy arising out of that assessment.

Disorders of articulation
Articulate speech involves selective, co-ordinated movements of the tongue, lips, jaw and soft palate, finely synchronised with direction of the air or sound stream. These movements modify the vocal tract in such a way that sounds of different nature, e.g. plosives, nasals, sibilants, can be produced. These sounds are the basis for the phonological system which is, in turn, basic to spoken language.

Disorders of articulation may arise from an inability to produce the requisite movements, or from inability to hear or to perceive the sounds with which those movements are associated. They may also arise from structural abnormalities which do not allow appropriate modifications of the sound wave. A mild defect of articulation may involve the faulty production of a sound so that attention is distracted but communication unimpaired. A severe disorder of articulation may render a person unintelligible because his phonological system is too restricted or too unstable for the linguistic weight which it has to carry.

Disorders of language

A disorder of language reflects the incomplete mastery of the linguistic or symbolic system common to the society. Causes must be looked for in the ability to receive and organise auditory and visual patterns, and in the ability to conform to the behaviour conventional to the society. A language disorder may be developmental, reflecting a discrepancy between the standards required by the society and the degree of accomplishment reached by a slowly maturing child.

Language disorder associated with hearing loss

The speech therapist will be employed in teaching and stimulating language and in teaching articulatory placement based on phonetic principles.

Language disorder associated with brain damage

The speech therapist is concerned with language stimulation, and with the pre-linguistic skills of attention, listening and signalling. She is later concerned with language teaching in all its aspects and throughout the general management.

Language disorder associated with mental retardation

The speech therapist will carry out language teaching and stimulation programmes in both E.S.N. and S.S.N. populations, but will also work to correct defective articulation and improve vocal quality and fluency.

Emotional disturbance

The speech therapist may be used to develop communication through language and to stimulate and teach language where this is perceived as being central to the child's communication disorder.

Disorders of fluency
Non-fluency; cluttering; stammering (stuttering)

Loss or partial breakdown of voice, speech and language:

1. Aphonia/dysphonia: Loss or partial loss of voice due to disease or injury to the larynx or its nerve supply. The cause may also be functional, involving misuse of the voice or personality maladjustment.
2. Anarthria/dysarthria: Loss or impairment of articulation of neuropathological origin.
3. Aphasia/dysphasia: Loss or partial loss of language following cerebral catastrophe.

When the Committee of Enquiry reported, it too used a broadly descriptive framework with the initial headings (3.07 – 3.30)

Disorders of voicing
Disorders of rhythm (stammering, stuttering)
Disorders of articulation
1. Specific developmental delay
2. Structural dysarthria
3. Neurological dysarthria
Disorders of language
1. Specific developmental delay
2. Acquired brain damage
3. Associated with hearing impairment
4. Associated with mental handicap
5. Associated with autism or psychoses
6. Associated with severe social deprivation

Mixed disorders

These headings are expanded and some further terms introduced. However the report itself strongly urges the need for and establishment of 'a universally accepted and understood system of classification of speech disorders and of defined criteria of defective speech' (10.12).

The only other classification to be offered by a member of the Committee is that of Ingram, publishing independently in the same year but in another connection (ed. Rutter and Martin, 1972). Ingram starts his chapter on 'The classification of speech and language disorders in young children' by saying that 'disorders of speech should be classified according to linguistic and phonetic criteria'. However, he is forced to concede that this is not at the moment possible and so opines that a 'classification based on the major functions of speech which is disordered and associated clinical findings is justifiable for practical purposes'. His ensuing classification presents a compromise between clinical manifestation and causation.

By the early seventies we then had broad categories of conditions with the choice made on pragmatic grounds; associated with these broad classifications were terms of varying degrees of specificity accepted with varying degrees of concurrence. The position in England was now moving from the earlier influence of European thinking, active during the college's first essays into terminology, to the much more pronounced influence of the United States. The major tests of speech pathology were coming from that country and its terminology was starting to have its effect. In 1971 the important handbook *Speech Pathology and Audiology* was revised under the editorship of Lee Edward Travis and the first chapter was devoted to terminology and nomenclature (Wood, 1971). That author in his introductory section suggests that 'if the student will acquaint himself with some of the Greek and Latin roots, prefixes and suffixes, he may be able to formulate central meanings of many terms even though the current meanings may have twisted away from the significance of the roots.' It will be apparent that this author does not altogether share Professor Wood's faith in this endeavour. Other statements open to challenge are those advocating an unbridled eclecticism in the vocabulary of speech pathology and therapy as this may not be reconcilable, to the student, with the dedication towards developing that technical vocabulary which 'is of signal importance'. Signs of the existing eclecticism are nicely revealed by glancing at the first four terms appearing under the letter 'b': 'babbling; baby-talk; barbaralia; basal ganglia.'

1. 'Babbling: A stage in the acquisition of speech during which the child carried on vocal play with its random production of different speech sounds.'

A familiar and well-loved term with a clear definition, but we cannot now assume that only one activity is contained within the term. Cruttenden writing in 1979 sets out the two suggested functions of babbling and reminds us also of the phenomenon of 'babbling drift.'

2. 'Baby-talk: A speech defect characterised by substitution of speech sounds similar to those used by the normal speaking child in the early stages of speech development. Same as *lalling* and *infantile speech*.'

This invites challenge on many points and would be unlikely to be used by any speech therapist or linguist. Its usefulness is therefore not to the professions concerned with communication but to parents and other interested lay people.

3. 'Barbaralia: Habitual use of the speech sounds and rhythmomelody of a native language while learning to speak another'.

A very pleasing term but, to this author's knowledge, never one in general use. To introduce it would be to invite cries of 'pejorative' since the word 'barbarian' is generally misconstrued. It might also, to those whose study of Greek is less than devoted, suggest only the common language of a number of females of the same name.

4. 'Basal ganglia: The collection or mass of nerve cells below the cortex of the brain connecting the cerebrum with the lower centres and comprising the thalami, corpora striata, corpora quadrigemina tuber cinerum and geniculate bodies.'

Here we may place some trust in constancy and certainty. It is not easy for a student of the subject to reconcile a technical vocabulary which contains such very simple terms as 'babbling' but might at any moment be asked to embrace 'gnosogenic dysautomaticity'. This last term was not cited by Professor Wood but is used by Mysak (1976) in his attempt to categorise speech pathologies by systems. Neither is it easy when the terms are used differently in the texts of two countries. Wood defines 'dyslalia' as 'defective articulation due to faulty learning or due to abnormality of the external speech organs and not to lesions of the central nervous system.' In Britain the term 'dyslalia' was never used for organically based conditions and only the first and last parts of Wood's definition would apply. It is not proposed that students should now take this terminological divergence too seriously since the term is not likely to be in use in the future. It was originally much favoured by speech therapists and in this country was sub-divided for clarity into the following:

Simple dyslalia: One sound or pair of sounds only affected

Multiple dyslalia: Several sounds affected

General dyslalia: Grammar affected in addition to articulation

The decline of the term came about in this way:

1. Speech therapists, finding the use of one term for many conditions and causes to be unhelpful, started to make their own accomodations. 'Dyslalia' was generally reserved for the main group with multiple sound substitutions. Where only one sound was involved the condition was either called by the Greek name for that sound 'sigmatism' 'rhotacism' or referred to as a simple speech defect. The groups were also found to be unsatisfactory in giving no clue as to causation and so requiring the ponderous 'associated

with mental retardation' or 'associated with emotional immaturity' to be added. This led to the replacement of the term by general descriptions on the one hand or more specific appellations on the other.

2. Speech therapists started to draw attention to conditions which showed some of the same type of behaviour as in dyslalia but which demanded a different approach. A major example comes from Morley's launching of the term 'apraxia' in the late 1950s, as cited in Chapter 3, page 40. Morley considered that a condition existed hitherto treated under dyslalia and involving sound substitutions and distortions. However, as the underlying basis was very different in this newly-demarcated condition, Morley and others believed that it would be clinically as well as academically improper to group them together. Thus with the detachment of those speech disorders associated with motor planning, dyslalia became further impoverished.

3. Speech pathologists writing from the U.S. offered other terms for the conditions covered by dyslalia, e.g. 'infantile perseveration' and 'delayed speech'. Also the widely used 'articulatory disorder' offered severe competition through the writing of, among others, Van Riper and Irwin (1958).

4. Other professions offered insights into the conditions affecting speech acquisition which lead speech therapists to review their own considerations. The significant work here was that presented by Grady and colleagues at the National Conference of 1962 and subsequently published (Grady, 1963). This drew on the work of Haas and showed a major influence by the subject which was from then on to dominate the field of childhood speech disorders – linguistics.

5. With the emergence of linguistics to engender theories of language breakdown and to describe the data in different ways, the kiss of death was given to dyslalia as a term. Among interested linguists, Smith, (1974) and Grunwell, (1976) writing in the British Journal of Disorders of Communication offered alternatives which were not only of theoretical interest but were helpful in working out methods of therapy. This proved conclusive.

In looking at the College's recommended vocabulary we see that terms may be considered to be helpful at one time and then rejected. This is not entirely a question of fashion although it plays some part. The implication is that more has been found out about the condition. Alternatively, a new theory may have been propounded which requires a new vocabulary. It is of interest to consider the terms that could have been used for the speech of the child William, cited in Chapter 2, depending on who was defining the conditon and when the definition was offered:

Hottentotism: The Hottentots were members of a South African tribe distinguished by their short stature and inferior intellect (the latter characteristic possibly unfair to Hottentots and certainly unfair to William)

Idioglossia: A personal tongue, separate and individual

General dyslalia

Expressive language disorder

Articulatory disorder

Phonological disability.

The first term Hottentotism would today be considered pejorative as is Mongolism. It is not very helpful in planning treatment since the actual language pattern is not described. If it were associated with a clearly defined syndrome clinicians would know what to expect and thence how to proceed.

Idioglossia suggests a unique language. Investigation would then be necessary to find out the nature of that language. Does the unique quality lie in the sound structures or in the use of words to convey thoughts? If the sounds are affected is it because they are abnormally produced or used differently? Again however, if there were general agreement on these points the word could indicate a recognisable condition and be associated with an approach to treatment.

The evolution and dissolution of the term dyslalia has already been discussed. In effect, the term would have suggested to prac-tioners at the time of its use that the child had no organic disability but that he needed help in mastering the salient features of spoken language. 'Expressive language disorder' takes us back into the category of broad description since we cannot determine from it which are the areas of language that need remedy. The next term 'articulatory disorder' draws attention to the production of sound patterns but is in danger of placing emphasis upon the mechanics of that production. The final term 'phonological disability' specifies the nature of the disorder. It indicates that the systemic element of sound use is at fault. We might therefore expect the child to be able to produce sounds but not to use them in the conventional way. We still have very limited information in that we do not know whether the condition is associated with pathology. Certainly no pathology is implied but we do not yet have agreement which states that phonological disabilities always arise from discriminatory problems or faulty learning.

We appear to be in a position to pinpoint areas of weakness, to describe them in linguistic terms and to demonstrate some of the pathologies which may give rise to them, but we have no technical vocabulary which comprehends both linguistic and medical phenomena. This alliance is approached in our definitions of acquired aphasia. Neurologists working with aphasic patients have had to make use of psycho-linguistic terms as they seek to describe the nature of the language deficit which arises from the neuropathology, but in this field the technical vocabulary is dominated by rival individuals or schools who have evolved their own amalgam or system of labels. There is a considerable range or diversity of opinion as to how to describe phenomena which all clinicians observe.

In other conditions where aetiological factors are more restricted and symptoms less diverse, we find less variation in terminology. The basic terms aphonia and dysphonia need less modification than do aphasia and dysphasia. This is simply to state that disorders of voice are less complex than those of language, but if we set out to establish the precise nature of the vocal impairment, we find ourselves in territory as uncharted as any other in the communication field. Laver's paper in the British Journal of Disorders of Communication (Laver, 1968) drew attention to the lack of definition, or even of basic agreement as to the ways to describe voice quality. Wynter and Martin in recent research have attempted to find a measure of agreement from judges which would allow for a classification of vocal disorders. This developed from a pilot project (Wynter, 1974) which again revealed the lack of agreement among therapists as to degrees of vocal divergence. If people cannot agree about states it is difficult to persuade them to agree about terms.

Disorders of voice, or voicing yield an important sub-category, that of resonance (Committee of Enquiry, 3.11). Disorders of resonance have suffered from the same terminological disadvantages as those of voice. Labels are easily found for conditions, e.g. hyperhinophonia, hyporhinolalia, but the conditions themselves are by no means clearly defined. Excessive nasal tone which is not grossly pathological is difficult to quantify. Objective measures can be made of degree and kind of palatal functioning but not of the adverse ratio of nasal to oral tone. The development of instrumentation may possibly allow these measures to be made soon. Some 20 years ago Renfrew, Mitchell and Wallace, three very experienced therapists, decided to objectify their criteria for nasality and started by rating patients independently. In spite of their high level of clinical experience and the experience they had shared as a therapeutic team, there was considerable divergence in their ratings. There is no reason to believe that any other therapeutic team would show a higher level of agreement. Judgement of tone quality is likely to remain extremely subjective in spite of instrumental measures.

The effect of excessive nasality may be given by abnormally limited articulatory movements and jaw opening. The relationship between one speech characteristic and another is very close. Where disorders cross boundaries and constitute a recognisable syndrome they may be called by the name of the syndrome. An example is 'cleft palate speech' which comprehends abnormal resonance and impaired articulation. Such a term is more meaningful to most speech therapists than the recently resurrected 'structural dysarthria' and is more convenient than the laborious 'hyperhinophonia associated with cleft palate'.

Similarly the term 'laryngectomised' is frequently used in speech therapy to refer, not simply to the operation, but to the ensuing voicelessness. To refer to patients who have suffered this condition as 'aphonic' is not appropriate. Nor is 'dysphonia' appropriate to their later state of vocal rehabilitation. 'Psuedo voice' though less elegant is more helpful.

Three of the four categories voice, articulation, and language and have shown themselves to embrace many conditions. The final one, fluency, suffered a change of name at the hands of the Committee of Enquiry (3.12) but is recognised by the profession to contain the major disorder of stammering (Dalton and Hardcastle, 1977). This disorder, however, is not one entity. It covers a very considerable range of speech behaviour from the evasive circumlocutions of the experienced avoider to the prolongations and repetitions of the child who lacks verbal proficiency. Neither can many kinds of stammering be properly described as disorders of speech since many stammerers speak normally as often as they stammer. This is a wide ranging condition of varying aetiology which may stem from, or be perpetuated by, personality difficulties. All current methods of treating stammerers make use of personality inventories and explore situational and social demands.

Non-fluent speech arises from severe discrepancies between different elements: content and formulation, vocabulary and articulation, communicative need and anxiety or inhibition. These discrepancies become paramount when there is pressure upon the speaker and the stammering behaviour is exacerbated by the reactions of other people. Different aspects of communicative deficiency are high-lighted by different situations. Those speakers whose lack of fluency is not strongly associated with anxiety may suffer less from personality difficulties than from poorly formulated utterance. There is likely to be a number of speakers in any speech therapy department with major difficulties of speech and prosody regulation. Here the onus may be placed upon defective monitoring rather than defective utterance. Thus the classifying focus shifts and the condition may be placed under language disorder since it is essentially founded in linguistic imbalance (for discussion of central language imbalance see Luchsinger and Arnold, 1965).

The discussion so far shows some of the difficulties that are found if a hard and fast terminology is devised to cover conditions which are not always fully understood and which are continually being re-explored. As information on the conditions is coming in from many different sources, the speech therapy student will need considerable guidance in acquiring an appropriate vocabulary to handle it. Practice among teaching departments will vary with regard to the introduction of speech therapy terms. Some strongly vocational departments will teach the students the technical vocabulary of their own subject before they are exposed to any other. Other instructors, who see speech pathology and therapy as evolving from a number of other disciplines, will propagate it after the student has studied the basic subjects. These subjects are likely to be anatomy, audiology, linguistics, phonetics, physiology and psychology. Some of these employ a consistent vocabulary with a tradition of use well established in the literature. Others use a broad array of terms some of which are words current in the normal language coinage but here given a specialised connotation. These will be more confusing to the student than will be the less familiar but arbitrarily established vocabularies of older subjects.

There are other terminological hazards for the student. One of these, and a major one, is the proliferation of jargon now occurring in every subject but particularly in the social sciences. The United States must unfortunately be held responsible for much of this proliferation in speech pathology. In seeking to express new concepts or to find new ways of describing old ones, language is used to obfuscate rather than to illuminate.

It cannot be stressed often enough that the purpose of a technical language is to express meaning clearly to colleagues not wilfully to disguise it from other people. It is particularly important for the speech therapist to appreciate this since she shares aspects of her work with members of many different professions and with non-professional workers. Such a broad and varied group cannot be expected to share a common technical language. The speech therapist must therefore understand the nature of the conditions with which she is dealing and so be able to explain them in clear and straightforward English. The specific terms used in professional reports to colleagues and in the literature should help her to understand the nature of those conditions by defining their major elements.

We will now consider the term *aphasia* within the discussion so far and within the context of the medical, developmental and language models described in Chapter 1. Aphasia has been described in a variety of professional and non-professional literature for many hundreds of years. A vivid account of a transitory episode was given by Dr Samuel Johnson and many textbooks on neurology refer to accounts by sufferers of their experiences. All these of course refer to the acquired condition. The use of the term for interference with developing language is much more recent. It is also strongly contested when it is used descriptively for behaviour rather than diagnostically when there is known brain damage.

Among the very many definitions of aphasia we will choose one of the broadest (Halpern, 1972). 'Aphasia may be defined as a multi-modality language disturbance due to brain injury'. 'It is a linguistic deficit that causes the individual to have difficulty in the comprehension and solidus or formulation of language symbols. Aphasia is not generalised intellectual impairment, apraxia of speech, confused language, or dysarthria, although components of any combination of those disorders may accompany aphasic disturbance'. Halpern is here writing about the acquired condition in adults and goes on, as do most writers on the subject to consider the different manifestations of aphasic disturbance and the different terms used for them.

Zangwill, in his introductory paragraph on 'The Concept of Developmental Dysphasia' (1978) approaches the condition in the same way. 'The term developmental dysphasia has come into general use to denote slow, limited or otherwise faulty development of language in children who do not otherwise give evidence of gross neurological or psychiatric disability. Accordingly, children with infantile hemiplegia or other forms of cerebral palsy are not normally classed as cases of developmental aphasia, even though their speech may be slow to develop and present various types of abnormality. Much the same is true of mentally handicapped or autistic children. In general, lack or impairment of speech secondary to deafness is likewise excluded from the category of developmental dysphasia, though it should be borne in mind that some degree of auditory defect, in particular high frequency deafness, may be found in some children who have been diagnosed as aphasic. On the whole, however, it may be said that the outstanding handicap of developmental dysphasia is social and educational rather than physical and that sensory and motor defects of any severity are seldom in evidence.'

Zangwill, having given this extremely cautious description then goes on to refer to other writers for evidence as to what aphasia is. He reminds us of Ewing's original work to affix childhood language disorders including aphasia within the framework of 'cerebral immaturity' or 'development lag'. He also refers to more recent literature indicating differences in brain function between the dysphasic child and other populations. The book containing Zangwill's chapter, *Developmental Dysphasia* edited by Maria Wyke, may be recommended as a good example of representatives of different disciplines attempting to discover the nature of a disability by examining different aspects of its manifestation.

Both Halpern and Zangwill could be challenged for being too wordy and for saying what aphasia is not rather than what it is. Eisenson, writing in 1968 is no more succinct. 'An aphasic child is one with central nervous system dysfunction. This dysfunction, which is presumably caused either by a failure or lag in cerebral maturation or because of cerebral damage, produces perceptual impairment that is associated with severe difficulty in the normal acquisition of language.' Eisenson then goes on to list the linguistic and behavioural manifestations that distinguish the child from other children.

We may therefore say that there is agreement that a condition of aphasia exists in an acquired form in adults and that there are established ways by which neurologists and others may arrive at a diagnosis of aphasia though there may be some disagreement as to how the term should be qualified in individual cases. We may also say that there is some agreement that developmental conditions in children, where there are severe difficulties in acquiring language and some evidence of interference with normal cortical function, may also be thus diagnosed. The common ground between the acquired and developmental conditions is:

1. Language impairment: in the one population, loss and in the other, faulty acquisition
2. Interference with normal cortical function: either demonstrated by neurological examination and brain scan or deduced from other symptoms.

Aphasia, as a term has therefore considerable utility and students should not be daunted by the apparent contradictions in the literature. It is likely too that experiments now being carried out into among other things, sound sequencing (Kracke, 1975) and auditory processing (Tallal and Piercy, 1978) will generate tests which will allow for positive identification.

The child cited in Chapter 1 (p. 11) will be seen as a suitable illustration of the above. It was seen that while medical investigation and developmental profile were helpful in drawing attention to areas of interest, the language model was more helpful to the therapist in checking performance and coming to a conclusion. Students would probably benefit from looking at conditions against such a model and trying to see what are the components of the condition which generate a technical term and what are their near neighbours in the whole area of linguistic function. Please refer to the bibliography of this Chapter for fuller reference.

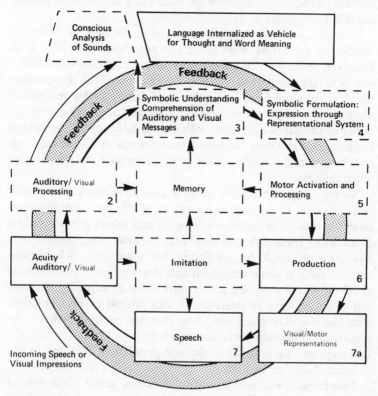

Fig. 2 (repeat)

1. Acuity

Interference with acuity will affect the whole process of language, comprehension, formulation and use, if congenital and severe. It is therefore appropriate to think in terms of the nature and severity of the loss. There are no terms in general use for phonological or syntactic reduction consequent upon hearing loss though these may well be postulated at some time.

2. Auditory processing

Interference here will cause confusion, both psychological and linguistic. If the former is severe much inhibition may be shown. Terms that are used here attempt to show which element is the most important.

Auditory agnosia: Inability to abstract meaning from sound
Congenital auditory imperception: Difficulty in perceiving the meaning of auditory imput
Congenital word deafness: Difficulty in associating words with meaning
Receptive aphasia: Inability to abstract meaning from speech
Receptive dysphasia: Difficulty in comprehending speech.

As auditory processing is shown as relating to symbolic understanding and memory any impairment here will lead to comprehension, storage and retrieval problems and will thus be reflected in the nature of the utterance. Word finding difficulty and verbal and literal paraphasia are thus strongly associated with auditory processing difficulty.

3. Symbolic understanding

Deficiencies in this area are related to disorders of cognition. Terms may therefore be drawn from psychology

Amentia: Absence or loss of intellectual function
Dementia: Disturbance of mental function
Mental retardation: Failure of intellectual development

If the deficiency is related to the one modality only, the resulting disability will be aphasia verbal asymbolia or visual agnosia or visual asymbolia. Autism is placed by some writers near to aphasia; by others within the category of dementia.

4. Symbolic formulation

Deficiencies or impairments of this process will result in inability to put thoughts into words or other symbols. It may be termed verbal asymbolia if there is an inability to comprehend verbal symbols in the first instance. If the disorder is confined to formulation it may be termed:

Expressive a/dysphasia
Executive a/dysphasia
Expressive language disorder.

5. Motor activation and processing

Deficiencies in this area will result in inability to take the verbal symbol or word through the stages of assembly which will allow it to be produced normally. Terms used by different writers indicate the stage of breakdown:

Aphemia: Loss of kinaesthetic word image

Apraxia for speech: Inability to produce speech sounds volitionally

Verbal a/dyspraxia: Inability to produce or imitate words accurately

Articulatory a/dyspraxia: Inability to produce or imitate sounds accurately.

It may be seen that not only do stages 2, 3, 4 and 5 relate to and influence each other but they all relate to memory. If there is interference with auditory memory stages 2 and 3 will be affected and ultimately 7; if visual memory is poor stage 3 and eventually stage 7a. If there is interference with kinaesthetic memory stages 5, 6, 7 and 7a will be affected. There may also be specific word finding difficulties which are directly related to memory.

It is therefore possible to have a patient with verbal dyspraxia and dysphasia if there has been damage to the neurological processes which underpin both functions. Similarly there may be mixed dysphasia, with both comprehension and formulation affected. If neurological damage is widespread, or if there is lack of brain growth and differentiation many symptoms will co-exist.

6. Production

Impairments here are likely to be classified according to the organ involved. If there is failure of laryngeal innervation or some structural abnormality of the larynx there will be:

Aphonia: Absence of phonation

Dysphonia: Impairment of phonation.

This will be qualified by descriptive or aetiological criteria (see earlier discussion). Faulty innervation or impaired structure may give rise to:

Anarthria: Absence of articulate speech

Dysarthria: Impairment of articulate speech

Stammering.

The earlier discussion has shown that the terms stammering may be appropriately related to impaired auditory or motor processing and to discrepancies between formulation and memory, but some research (Wyke, 1969) suggests that the initial interference in stammering can come from vocal spasm of neurological origin.

When students are confronted with terms that they do not fully understand they should seek to work them out:

1. From the root of the term
2. From the context in which it is used
3. By looking at it within some such scheme or representation as has been indicated here.

If students are in doubt as to what term to use they should:

1. Select the one that indicates most clearly the nature of the condition
2. Use the simplest term if it conveys meaning adequately
3. Give a brief definition of the term being used within the general description of the condition.

With cases where there are changes to be expected, it may be necessary to combine clear description with technical terms. For example global aphasia, in which the patient shows no real use of speech nor comprehends much of it, may give place to a condition where verbal formulation is the major deficit. It is helpful to record this process by indicating the improvement in comprehension rather than by simply exchanging one term for another.

The conditions which small children present do not easily lend themselves to rigid classification. It is for this reason that it is at present fashionable to refer to delayed speech or deviant speech in the first instance. These conditions have been described by the author as follows (Byers Brown, 1974):

'Delayed speech involves the late appearance of words and their combination into phrases and sentences. Rudimentary utterance and general behaviour may be on normal lines but the speech is less mature and less accomplished than is considered appropriate for the child's age or is common among his peers. The utterance would be suitable to a younger child and could be found in the normal developmental sequence. The delay may be apparent in the phonology, syntax or in the child's use of speech to control his environment. Deviant speech does not fit into a normal developmental sequence. It may manifest itself in voice or tone quality, sound structure or sound sequence. While gross deviations are likely to be associated with pathology, deviant phonological or syntactical constructions can occur in the absence of pathology, suggesting that the child is having difficulty in making deductions from the stream of sound he hears or that he is not able to make use of his deductions to build up his language system in a conventional manner.'

This same paper offers discussion of several terms used interchangeably with delayed speech. Many such terms will doubtless continue to be offered, emphasis being placed by different authors on the element perceived to be particularly vulnerable or at fault. Linguists now moving into this field are adding to the number of ways of describing the conditions encountered, but they are unlikely to cause the same confusion in students' minds as do the terms of speech pathology because they are rooted in concepts already taught in normal language acquisition and functions. The people to recoil from linguistic terminology will be the established practitioners who did not learn these tools and vocabulary during their training. Fortunately they too are well served by literature and by the willingness of many linguists to co-operate in clinical discussions.

While the linguistic terminology is likely to establish itself rather firmly in the immediate future it would be, in the opinion of the author, a mistake to throw out the medical terms. As has been indicated in preceding chapters, we are now seeing the start of a much cheaper and accessible technology. New ways of assessing physiological properties could reverse the move to describe function in behavioural terms. The student is wise therefore to tolerate a state of creative doubt in this area, as in so many others, and to make unashamed compromise between terminological demands if she sees it as being the most helpful way to describe the condition.

Many neurologically impaired children show disorders of language and articulation. Thus dysphasia, dyspraxia and dysarthria may be encountered at different times and simultaneously. The following are extracts taken from reports sent to medical officers and teachers who had the children in their care. In both instances there is attempt to describe the nature of the condition and suggest what should be done to assist the child. They are not offered as models for report writing but rather to show how technical terms may have to be combined with non-technical information. They therefore illustrate something of the nature of terminological compromise.

Case report: Joan aged 4 years 11 months
Joan's habitual expression was open mouthed with drooping lower lip. Her facial muscles appeared somewhat flaccid and her face expressionless unless animated by lively play. She was able to perform movements of smiling, frowning and lip pursing but her face lacked the change of movement of the normal child. She was unable to maintain lip closure and appeared to have to make an effort to hold her lips together even for a short time. Her lower jaw lies forward in relation to the upper (as does her mother's) and she

shows an edge to edge bite with an open space between the incisors. Her tongue habitually protrudes between her teeth. I did not notice much movement of the tongue when she was concentrating on an activity. There seemed to be no active sucking or thrusting behaviour only the rather inert forward fall of the tongue.

Joan was able to direct air forward for gentle but sustained blowing, rounding her lips in the process. I was unable to obtain a view of the soft palate upon oral examination because the tongue was retracted up and back. The hard palate is very high and narrow as is often found in children with abnormal tongue posture. Joan could protrude and retract her tongue voluntarily and move it around a little, but during laughter and some speech attempt it was retracted back so that the tip broadened out and the frenum was prominent..

Sample words were produced rather tentatively. They were uttered in a husky voice with break between vowel and consonant. As the session continued they were pronounced with more assurance and clarity. Words included:

day-i	daddy	me	
do	dog	tu	come
baw	ball	clo	clock
car			
mummy			

The quality of the words varied but it was noticeable that under strong stimulation speech become much clearer. It appears that there is a strong factor of inhibition here and the little girl will not, or cannot, attempt an utterance unless it is familiar or unless very strongly motivated.

All my observations suggest that Joan has a severe language disorder and is in immediate need of speech therapy and special education. Further observation and assessment will delineate the areas of strength and weakness more clearly but all aspects of language functions are involved.

I believe that the lack of movement of the speech organs and their reduced proprioceptive sensation are a major factor. The little girl has not been able to experiment in sound play nor to make the normal connections between utterance, repetition, imitation and the reception and perception of sound sequences.

I would suggest that she be put on an immediate programme designed to increase the number of her utterances in order to give her more oral sensation and control. The words that she can say she should be encouraged to say with increased speed and varied volume so that she gains more control. Sounds now available to her should be practiced at speed and humming sounds combined with vowels in different intonation patterns to increase length and tone.

I would regard these motor skills as very important but they should be combined with language stimulation to improve comprehension and memory. Although her mother talks to Joan as much as she can, a speechless child very rarely receives as much language stimulation as a normal child. Her inability to ask 'why' and 'what for' mean that she is rarely given the kind of explanation necessary for normal linguistic growth.'

Case report: Katy aged 6 years.

'The following suggestions are made on the assumption that Katy's speech has not developed normally because she has not been able to make and co-ordinate the movements appropriate for articulate utterance. We are therefore seeing a specific dysarthria or articulatory difficulty of structural/neurological origin coupled with a general retardation of language.

Language: We suggest that this be helped by simple story telling, encouraging Katy to listen to stories which have repetition and that the length of the stories be greatly increased. It would also be helpful to make up a story for her with picture cards so that she can concentrate on listening to a sentence at a time while looking at a picture. Games involving sequences, counting and naming should be encouraged to help memory. Discrimination of words and sounds should be practised with appropriate emphasis and/or accompanying gesture, e.g.

This is an old cat
This is a cold cat
This is an old hat.

Katy needs to be helped to appreciate sound changes. She is not able to make these herself yet, but she may begin to do so.

Speech. Katy needs a more normal basis of movement and sound play on which to build the sounds of speech. She has not passed through all the early vocalising and babbling activity of normal infants, nor has she exercised the speech organs through normal sucking, chewing and swallowing. It is not suggested that she be put back to these earlier stages, but rather that they be incorporated as far as possible with her present speech development procedures. The following activities may be useful:

1. Chewing, pursing and kissing movements of the lips
2. Combining the above with vocalising so that patterns of babbling and sound play emerge

3. Encouraging Katy to vocalise and babble with different intonation. Play 'echo' with one person producing sounds, e.g. 'OO-ee' (as in 'Coo-ee') and the other one copying. Be sure to keep these sounds within the normal range
4. Encourage humming and use lip plucking or additional vibration (comb and paper) to promote sensation
5. Add 'l' 'l' to vocalising so that 'la' 'la' is formed
6. Then practise calling 'hallo'
7. Build up to 'hallo mummy' – 'who's there?' 'me' so that meaningful words and phrases are built up on the most normal flowing sounds possible.

It is appreciated that Katy will continue to use her present speech pattern which involves glottal stops, vowels and stress for some time to come in general communication. This has arisen because she has not been able to build up air pressure and produce appropriate consonants at the level of lips and front or back of tongue, so she has been forced to use such sounds as she can generate and control to convey meaning. We hope that these will gradually give way to a more normal pattern of utterance as she becomes more competent but the change over will naturally be slow.

We all believe it to be in Katy's interests that she be encouraged to communicate and express herself as freely as possible. Suggestions made for altering the speech pattern are therefore made with this general premise in mind.'

As more expertise is shared between medical and educational workers (Warnock, 1978) it may be possible for professional people to communicate more immediately and succinctly. It will remain the responsibility of the speech therapist however to ensure that the condition she is treating is fully understood by her and by her colleagues and that this understanding generates the labels that are used.

Speech therapy in practice

SECTION TWO

Speech therapy in practice

7

Delays and disorders in developing speech — (1)

CONDITIONS WHICH ARE PATHOLOGICALLY BASED

Children may be born with structural or neurological abnormalities which make it impossible for them to acquire speech in the normal manner. If the structural abnormality is immediately apparent steps will be taken to treat the infant surgically or by prosthesis so that when he starts to speak he will already have been given improved equipment for the process. In other children the defect is not apparent until the child starts to speak abnormally. In cases of mild neurological disorder the child may not appear to have a handicap until the speech fails to develop normally. This failure will promote investigation which may reveal the pathology. It is not uncommon for the less profound forms of mental retardation to be masked until there is delay in developing speech. So in many cases the therapist may meet the child for the first time when he has already started to develop his own strategy to cope with his handicap or to avoid its consequences.

The involvement of speech therapists in guidance and treatment of very young children means that assessment is being made and remedy prescribed while the child is developing and changing. The physiological and psychological systems that subserve speech are subject to growth and influence. The child will be experiencing new constraints and new opportunities and be adapting to a variety of demands while the therapist is trying to improve his communicative skills. Sometimes he may make an excellent accommodation without her aid. Sometimes he will be defeated by the increasing demands on his inadequate mechanism and be unable to move without her help. At other times he will develop strategies of self-help which are not bad in themselves and which may even be temporarily effective but which will prevent him moving along the mainstream of childhood accomplishments.

It has been continually emphasised that communication disorders arise from a combination of constitutional and environmental inadequacies. Children with deficiencies in their speech or hearing mechanism may be able to compensate very adequately or not at all depending on their other advantages. Studies in the early literature of speech therapy frequently draw attention to the predisposing and precipitating factors which must co-exist when disabilities develop out of handicaps. Whatever the handicap there will always be three factors which the speech therapist must consider:

1. The initial problem; its physical or psychological basis
2. The child's growth and strategies of self-help
3. The continuing influence of his environment.

It will be apparent from looking at the language model and reconsidering some of the points made in earlier chapters that some pathological conditions will have a much more pervasive effect on the whole language learning process than others (for further discussion of non-clinical and clinical categorisation see Bloom and Lahey, 1978).

Impaired auditory acuity or hearing loss

The speech therapist's responsibility in the identification of hearing loss is considerable and has already been indicated. Hearing loss is still the first factor to be considered in cases of delayed speech and the Quirk report (Committee of Enquiry, 1972) re-affirmed the importance of routine and skilled hearing testing for every speech impaired child. This will inevitably mean that some children are seen for testing who have no hearing difficulties whatsoever and whose parents stoutly affirm that they have never had any, but it is infinitely better to be sure. Experienced speech therapists believe themselves well equipped to decide whether or not a particular speech pattern indicates the presence of hearing loss. They may therefore retain some children for their own assessment and only refer to the audiologists those children whose hearing is suspect. Other speech therapists, exhorted to economise and to relieve the burden on over-worked audiologists, may postpone tests pending response to therapy. While these procedures can be justified they should not be recommended. They will dilute the concentration on the importance of hearing in young children and this has already suffered because of economies in services. Students in training must be taught the importance of proper hearing measures and must carry the message with them upon qualifying.

A sensible move is to have one speech therapist in an area specially trained in audiological work so that she can carry out the preliminary assessments if necessary and can act as a resource person for colleagues who have only a basic acquaintance with audiology. Hearing testing in young children is an extremely skilled task requiring constant practice. Any children who fail to pass the speech therapist's assessment must be referred or preferably taken by her to a central clinic or specialised centre where such testing is available.

When hearing loss has been diagnosed the speech therapist may join the team of those concerned with communication training. Her place on the team will depend upon her own expertise and interest. All speech therapists should be able to assist the mildly hearing-impaired child or the one whose loss can be relieved by surgery to improve his listening and speech skills. Many speech therapists are now specialising in work with severely deaf children. Children with significant hearing losses need the skilled help of teachers of the deaf. They may encounter these as infants, when the focus is on parent guidance; in schools for the hearing impaired; in units or on a peripatetic visiting basis if the child can attend normal school. The teacher of the deaf is responsible for the child's education and linguistic growth is the key to this.

The speech therapist contributes those particular elements of care for which she is best equipped. Her remit will be to assess and then, if necessary, to improve the comprehension and production of linguistic forms, prosody, phonology and syntax. These linguistic forms cannot be divorced from the content which generates them and gives them meaning. 'Children learn language to represent the information they know about events in the world – not as an empty signal to be discriminated, recalled in sequences, or pulled apart and put together again' (Bloom and Lahey, 1978). So the therapist must work closely with the teacher who has the child's daily language under surveillance and can take every opportunity to extend and re-inforce it. The speech therapist offers her detailed knowledge of language acquisition and her professional training in changing patterns of speech. She must apply herself to the speech of deaf children recognising that they may be unable to perceive the majority of those contrasts upon which normal language acquisition depends.

The deaf child lacks that sensory input to the brain which will allow him to develop language. If the hearing loss is partial he will receive some of the necessary input. We may see from his audiogram the extent of his problem of audition but that does not give sufficient guidance as to how to teach him. The important question is that of the relationship between reduced acuity and the perception of linguistic features and secondarily the effect of this perception upon production. It is because the relationship is so complex that the speech of the child cannot be deduced from his audiogram alone. There is a high degree of variation between the speech of children with essentially identical audiograms. It has effectively been demonstrated that the degree of hearing loss is the most important single factor affecting linguistic development and speech intelligibility (Markides, 1970), but individual aspects of the child's endowment must have their effect just as does his environment. So in attempting to help an individual child to improve his speech the therapist must carry out a detailed assessment of his utterance and of his comprehension and production of linguistic features. She must be trained to appreciate the possible effects of amplification upon the nature of these features.

The foci of therapy in cases of hearing impairment have been touched upon in Chapters 4 and 5. The child is blocked at the level of acuity and consequently the whole dependent process of perception, recognition and discrimination (processing) cannot operate. The child cannot take the first step towards language mastery because he is not receiving acoustic cues. Neither can he proceed to the next stage of language acquisition; that of verbal symbols or words. So his brain is not stimulated or activated to work out a system of language, using the input of others as the bricks for his individual construction. (For a very elegant exposition of this process see Fry, 1977 and 1978). If we apply the concept of rate determining reaction we will see that unless the acuity barrier can be overcome the child will build up energy at a non-linguistic level. He will fail to make use of linguistic cues and he will organize his behaviour from the environmental cues which he sees and believes to be significant. He will also persist in infantile pre-language activities because these are the only ones available to him.

The language learning of the hearing impaired child, arrested at the level of acuity, may be facilitated in the following ways:

1. Through the auditory channel
2. Through the auditory channel with strong visual support
3. Through the visual and motor channels with auditory support.

The choice will be made by the primary professional team of audiologist, teacher of the deaf and psychologist with the speech therapist contributing. The decision to rely mainly on auditory stimulation will depend not only upon the extent of the hearing loss but upon the suitability of the amplification that can be provided. It will also depend upon the child's intelligence and linguistic aptitude, the amount of stimulation and support he receives from his family and the availability of early parent guidance following early diagnosis. The teacher will still make very considerable use of vision, touch and movement in the development of linguistic concepts but will expect the child to be able to use auditory input, suitably amplified, to deduce the features of the linguistic system.

The speech therapist will not be involved in work with such children unless she is already attached to a unit where her contribution is regarded as routine. In this case she may assist the teacher by carrying out assessments at the phonological and syntactical level and generally giving input as to the child's progress. She owes this skill to the new tools of phonological and syntactical analysis developed by the linguists and will therefore share it with linguists and to some extent with teachers of the deaf. The last group is also equipping itself with the tools of syntactical analysis (see Crystal, Working with LARSP, 1979) but lacks the phonetic and phonological training which characterises the speech therapist.

Visual support

Until recently the main source of visual support to the child has been lip reading which has been of assistance only at sound and word production level. However, the development of visual display systems has given speech therapists and teachers a new means of demonstrating and enhancing those prosodic features which are the essential underpinnings of normal language and contribute so much to intelligibility. The work of Fourcin and Abberton has been paramount in this area. Speech therapy students are now being trained to use such systems with a variety of speech handicapped people who lack appropriate feedback. The systems have the outstanding advantage over other forms of support in that they are occurring in real time and give immediate feedback but can then allow patterns of speech to be held on the screen in visual form so that the child can continue to modify his production to bring it nearer to the model. As pointed out in Chapter 5, the proliferation of such aids is only just beginning but is likely to have a revolutionary effect upon all aspects of speech monitoring.

Visual and motor representations

The decision to use gesture and sign systems as the primary means of communication with the hearing impaired will again be made by the primary professional team. The speech therapist who is especially trained in the use of such systems may be of assistance to them. The decision will not only be whether to use such a system but when to use it. A case can be made for allowing the severely hearing impaired child to make his first systematic attempts at communication this way. A case can also be made for stimulating the auditory channel as much as possible and bringing in visual motor systems at a later date. The decisions that are made are extremely important ones for the child and his family and every effort should be made to reduce particular and professional partiality so that the interests of the child are the abiding focus and concern.

The hearing impaired population is outstandingly united by its main handicap. Compared to many other groups in the speech therapist's clinical population it may seem homogeneous, but it is of course made up of individuals with different talents, inheritances and dispositions. Within these will lie the possibility of linguistic problems independent of hearing loss. The child's particular linguistic strategies may make it difficult for him to learn through the methods selected to compensate for his hearing loss. There are factors of neurological maturation, cognition and motivation also to be considered. Throughout the normal population we find clumsy speakers and those with imprecise sound production. Because of their good hearing they can modify their speech and keep it within normal limits, but if the outstanding mentor is not available their small problems will not be controlled. They will in fact add to the speech production difficulty already in force because of hearing loss (Byers Brown, 1977).

Associated handicaps
The aetiology of deafness makes it likely that some forms will co-exist with structural and neurological impairments. Outstanding examples are cleft palate and cerebral palsy. There is also the group of neurologically impaired children whose receptive language disorders combine hearing loss and auditory imperception. All multiply handicapped children with communication problems are entitled to the care of the speech therapist in treatment as well as in diagnosis. Their treatment will be dominated by their major handicap and so the principle focus will vary. Even within the one child there may be a shift of treatment as certain handicaps are revealed as more problematic at a particular time. This point will be illustrated subsequently.

Having reviewed the nature and extent of the child's hearing problem and discussed his management with colleagues and parents the speech therapist will select those of her skills which are most helpful. It is likely that these will involve most of those suggested in Chapter 2.

Hearing impairment
Training foci:

Modifying behaviour
Training attention

If the child has been diagnosed early and received skilled parent guidance the essential modifications of behaviour will already have taken place. He will have learned to look at the speaker and his interest in sound and speech will have been aroused. He will be attracted towards verbal communication and he will associate it with his play. If his hearing loss has been diagnosed late and his parents have not received guidance these essential modifications will not have taken place. They must therefore be put into effect at once by all those dealing with the child. His behaviour must be controlled and he must be prepared for leaning.

The child's attention must be trained upon visual then auditory stimuli. The relationship between these two modalities must be established but the therapist should not forget the normal development sequence. The child may have to be led through the stages of distractability and rigidity that characterise early development and care must be taken not to place too many demands upon him, vital though his attention training is. The therapist must be attractive to the child and her speech lively and interesting.

Training listening
Training auditory discrimination and judgement

We are first concerned to bring to the child's awareness the nature and interest of speech. He needs to listen in the expectation that his listening will be rewarded. Vivid, simple speech which highlights interesting activities is indicated. Thus the child becomes aware of verbal contrasts and the differences between words. We are then concerned with training him to listen for contrasts in sounds so that he may acquire a systematic phonology. As this develops his listening may be focussed upon small morphological changes which govern meaning.

Training movement
Teaching control over patterns of movement

These are supportive skills which will come into play if the child is not able to proceed by auditory means. Attention can be drawn to articulatory placement. Movements of tip, blade, or back of the tongue can be highlighted by touch (tongue, blade or finger). Movements of the lips can be helped by the therapist actually putting them in position for the child and opening them lightly or pushing them forward. All movements must be associated with acoustic input and practised until they can be made swiftly enough to be integrated into the flowing utterance.

Teaching sequential skills

If these skills do not emerge in the child as the result of attention to amplified speech they may need highlighting through visual display. If profound difficulties are encountered a co-existent aphasic element may be present. In this case teacher and therapist will select a much more structured approach to all areas of language teaching with emphasis on the sequential relationships between sounds and words supported by considerable visual cueing.

Training imitation

This is likely to be an early focus of attention since it may be used in combination with all other skills. It is part of all techniques of matching and modelling and these are highly necessary to improve speech and expand language. Imitation may be required to be conscious if direct placement techniques are employed. It is also required as a conscious activity when using visual displays.

Teaching sound production

This has already been indicated in discussion of training movement. The child's speech flow may have to be slowed down to enable him to learn the production of any sound which is interfering with his intelligibility. We now think in terms of phonological rather than articulatory problems but both may exist. The deaf child is likely to show persisting constraints of vowel and consonant harmony. Certain features, e.g. retroflexion, may occur, dominated by certain sounds. The therapist may need to teach an alternative production of this sound and then use it to break up the overriding pattern.

If there is an articulatory defect, usually associated with motor control, the appropriate sound will need to be taught by visual, tactile and kinaesthetic means and re-inforced until used by the child. The relationship between production and perception is such that it may be necessary to interpolate this skill into the early stages of discrimination. Producing sounds will help children to form judgements about the structure of language.

Developing vocabulary

While this is highly necessary for hearing impaired children it is not a primary focus for the speech therapist. She must, of course, be aware of the child's severe deficiencies in this area and encourage vocabulary growth by using new words, well demonstrated and re-inforced, in her work with the child.

Teaching representational systems of expression

The contribution of the speech therapist has already been indicated. At the other end of the speech circuit are those mechanisms specifically concerned with speech production or the utterance of sound patterns. Damage or maldevelopment here means that sounds will be abnormally produced.

Abnormal sound production associated with faulty mechanism

Once again the first responsibility of the speech therapist will be the precise identification of difficulty. She will contribute her knowledge to the team lead by the paediatrician or plastic surgeon. Evidence from all aspects of oral behaviour will be put together to give the most complete picture possible of the state of the mechanism. To this must be added all other information about the child which will suggest how he can be helped to compensate. The speech therapist may be called upon to prepare the child for speech so that he may best benefit from an improved mechanism, or she may be required to help him achieve acceptable utterance when he has been given the mechanism. A third alternative will be to help him make a good accommodation in using a speech mechanism that can never be normal.

The therapist must draw on all the processes which are involved in speech to make a contribution to a better final result. Although the problem is apparently localized in the end organ, its control and compensation can only be achieved by attention to the whole process.

The child with a faulty speech mechanism lacks the ability to produce sounds by the conventional postures and movements of the articulators. If he attempts to make the same movements as other people the result will be different because he lacks appropriate contact points or valving mechanisms. If he adapts his movements because of acoustic information in order to achieve a better acoustic result, he will have to re-adapt if his mechanism is changed. It is of the greatest importance to the therapist to know exactly what the child is doing before she makes any attempt to intervene. Consequently investigations by endoscopic and radiological means must be pursued. These investigations are described in several of the books listed at the end of this chapter. Therapy may be carried on concurrently and will yield information that may generate further investigations.

Training foci:

Relaxation and control of posture

Children attempting to compensate for inadequate mechanisms will tend to set up a high degree of localised tension. An outstanding example is to be found in the tense and retracted tongue of the child with an incompetent naso-pharyngeal sphincter. Here the tongue takes up its abnormal posture to try to seal off the nasal cavity which is inadequately protected by the palatal action. A persisting movement of this kind will rob the tongue of much of its free and flexible activity during speech so that there is further sound distortion. A new movement cannot be built on an abnormal old one. First some relaxation of the tongue must be carried out. When it can take up a neutral position, there must be attention drawn to the accompanying tactile sensations so that the child has some guidance as to how to recapture the posture. Then new placements must be taught. These will bring into play a combination of visual and auditory impressions. At the very simplest level the therapist may say 'your tongue is lying very nicely in your mouth. Now look at yourself in the mirror while I say "la, la, la". Now lift your tongue and make the sound with me'. By this process the therapist makes a direct link at a basic level of control:

Auditory
Visual $\Big\}$ Acuity $\longrightarrow$ Imitation $\longrightarrow$ Production

If this is successful she will facilitate the link by repetition of the activity. Then she will raise the process to a more conscious level by bringing in:

Auditory discrimination and/or processing $\longrightarrow$ Memory $\longrightarrow$ Motor activation and processing

The child will start to take the responsibility for the appropriate production. The focus of training will then be upon:

Training movement
Training auditory discrimination and judgement
Training imitation
Teaching sound production.

This will, of course, constitute a constellation of behaviour modification processes so that suitable rewards will be built in by the therapist as required.

Invoking the next level of activity will bring in the whole linguistic and communicative aspects of speech. As is frequently found, the child who has only attained partial control at a lower level may break down when he has to re-order the movement within the linguistic framework, especially when dominated by enthusiasm. Here the therapist must decide how capable the child is of deducing for himself where the new behaviour is required. Generally speaking children with poor intelligence need much more time to consolidate any new behaviour and require a slower and more re-inforced movement forward than do intelligent children. But changing behaviour, particularly in a personal skill brings in attitudes as well as intelligence. The child is being asked to accept a different picture of himself and may need time to do this. Here, as always, mechanics and philosophy jostle each other for pride of place.

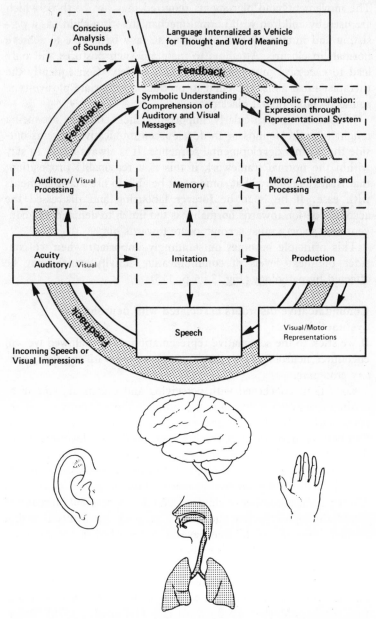

Fig. 3

The processes just described will be brought into play whatever the structural abnormality, but the specific movement and postures to be trained will depend upon the nature of the structural fault. The movements and placements required may not be those which are used by children with normal mechanisms. If a child has a persisting and immutable mal-occlusion he may be unable to achieve normal lip closure. Attempts to maintain such postures will only lead to excessive muscular tension and anxiety. Consequently the therapist must assist the child to produce appropriate plosive-type sound by labio-dental placement.

Judgement is particularly important when children are being taught to make sounds or to develop communicative systems outside the normal developmental sequence. It is always better to stay within the normal framework if this is a reasonable proposition; that is, if the child will at some point be able to use his attainments with ease. If he is to be forever labouring and distressed the accommodation towards normality is too much to demand and conventional society must accommodate towards him.

This principle becomes outstandingly important when we consider the next levels of communicative activity which may be affected by pathology (Fig. 3 on p. 115).

Communicative disorders associated with neurological dysfunction

If we stick to the schemative representation so far followed we will encounter neurological dysfunction associated with *impaired auditory processing*.

Conditions concerned with perceiving and organising stimuli as distinct from responding to it at a simple reflex or routine level are particularly difficult to diagnose. The speech therapist's contribution here is therefore considerably concerned with diagnosis. Children who do not respond normally to sound are most properly referred to the audiology clinic, but they do not necessarily emerge from it with the hypothesis of hearing loss confirmed or refuted. There will be a number of children who do not respond normally to sound although objective audiometry suggests that acuity is within normal limits. Such children have been described in the literature since the founding of hearing clinics (Ewing, 1930; Taylor, 1967). Other children show a reduction of acuity which cannot be held responsible for the full extent of abnormal function. These children may be tested again and again with inconclusive or even contradictory results, (Morley, 1973; Ward and McCartney, 1978). Reference has already been made to the unsatisfactory position of the diagnostic procedure in discussing child B in Chapter 3 and the nature of developmental aphasia in Chapter 6. It is to be hoped that more positive means of identification will come about possibly on the lines indicated by Kracke (1975), to replace the present position of diagnosis by negation.

Unlike the conditions associated with hearing or structural impairment, those associated with neurological dysfunction do not lend themselves to direct compensation or restitution and are unlikely to do so whatever improvement there is in diagnosis. The speech therapist accordingly works with a different team. Once a diagnosis has been postulated, even if not fully established she will take her place with the teacher and psychologist in a slow process of education. The educational placement of the child will depend on the severity of his condition and the extent of his other resources but the help offered is of an educative not curative nature.

Training foci:

Training attention

According to the developmental state and the severity of the impairment attention may be trained:

1. Through visual channels
2. Through visual channels with auditory support
3. Through auditory channels with visual support.

Reference has already been made to the important work of Dr Joan Reynell and the Wolfson team in defining procedures for these early stages, but however much progress may be made in the control of selective attention there will remain children with profound difficulty in maintaining attention to speech. The process of absorbing the important signals from data given at the speed of speech is too hard and too fatiguing. It is no use concentrating training at the attention level if it is breaking down because of the nature of the task. Neither is it any use concentrating the child's attention if the basis of his problem is inability to make an attentional shift.

Training auditory discrimination and judgement. Here the teacher and therapist are trying to break through into the auditory storage system.

Acuity $\longrightarrow$ Auditory processing $\longrightarrow$ Memory

If this can be achieved there is hope that higher levels of activity can then be brought into play to consolidate and extend language learning. If this cannot be achieved the child will build up energy at the acuity level to the extent that he will either become extremely distressed by sound or will cut it out and inhibit any response. To prevent this happening the team will switch to visual signs and activate visual motor representations. The attempt would still be made to break through to the storage areas and then to higher centres of symbolic function but the avenue would be different. Evidence has been offered that if this route is taken the child may be able to make more use of the auditory system at a later date. This is psychologically sound in that if frustration is relieved, function is improved, but its actual neurophysiological basis awaits elucidation.

Training sequential skills

Whatever the modality used, such training is at present seen to be essential for children who have processing difficulties. The failure to acquire a linguistic system is seen by many as a failure to cope with temporal sequences. Emphasis on order and pattern will be built into any educative programme with these children.

If the auditory processing disorders are mild the child may only present with difficulties at the linguistic stage. These may involve phonological and syntactic patterning. The child may show attentional fatigue because he has difficulty with processing auditory information at speed and this fatigue may cause semantic errors (for a delightful excursion into this area see Aitchison, 1972). Semantic errors also arise from faulty guessing because the child lacks ability to make full use of acoustic cues (Byers Brown, 1970). If the child has reached this stage the thrust of therapy may be linguistic rather than pre-linguistic. It may train the skills of judgement and selection by contrasting words and drawing attention to both meaning and structure.

Another group of *neurologically dysfunctioning* children will show a constellation of difficulties at the motor activation and processing stage. The neurological basis for this, as for auditory processing, cannot yet be definitively described and diagnosis may still be made by psychological as much as neurological examination. The child's good comprehension will disprove auditory processing and memory deficits and so the disorder must be presumed to lie between these skills and those of production. In spite of good understanding the child fails at the level of production and sound constancy. Such a child has been described by the author (1972 et sequor) and her condition treated and studied for many years. In this case the hypothesis was made that the failure was not in any one system but in the coupling of the auditory and motor systems. In other cases the difficulty may be more firmly in the area of sound formulation and once sound production is taught the child may make use of auditory control to monitor it. The training foci in these cases may therefore be concentrated on teaching sound production. This may have to start at a phonetic level if the difficulty is extreme. As soon as possible, however, the therapist will move on to a contrastive, phonological approach which will assist the child to worry out the nature of sound and words. An important decision in cases of this kind is whether to go for consonant/vowel imitation which will more easily be moved on to a word or whether to start by a consonant sound and steadily associate it with vowels using the blending method advocated by McGinnis (1963). The developmental, babble-type approach using consonant and vowel as one unit is much more popular now but needs are more important than fashions and opinions and if such approaches do not lead to sound constancy and control the more analytic method must be employed. The following training stages will be:

Teaching control over patterns of movement — associated with sound
Training imitation
Developing vocabulary.

Once more it will be seen that if the difficulty is profound there will be a considerable build up of energy at the stage where input should lead to output. It will be necessary to provide other emotional and expressive outlets for the child through play. It may also be desirable to teach an alternative system of communication to give the child encouragement and support while he is struggling to become verbal (for more comprehensive discussion of children with processing and symbolic difficulties see Cooper and Griffiths, 1978).

Another ill-defined group whose difficulties are considered to be associated with impaired motor processing is the apraxic one. Some of the problems of definition in this area have already been considered in Chapter 6. While debate on the definition is likely to continue it may be said that there is a group of children whose major difficulty is in regulating and planning movement and in following through a sequence of movements. These children have been described as within the 'clumsy child' syndrome (Walton et al, 1962). They continue to be discussed and described and at the present time considerable attention is being drawn to their poor proprioception and impaired body image. These are considered to have a pathological basis as the behaviour is far outside the normal range of clumsiness and the person is always vulnerable to breakdown in following a pattern of movement (see the case of Peter, cited in Chapter 1).

Speech is severely affected in some of these children at a sound and word level (Morley, 1972; Edwards, 1973). They are therefore the proper concern of the speech therapist and require specially adapted programmes of articulation and language development.

Training foci:

Training imitation

This is a very weak skill in such children and unless it is strengthened they cannot benefit from other techniques. The speech therapist should start with imitation of larger movements before moving down to speech postures. Considerable repetition should be employed to build up body image (for a helpful exposition here see Grimley and McKinlay, 1977).

Teaching sequential skills

Teaching control over patterns of movement.

These may be employed concurrently as they assist each other.

Teaching sound production

This should follow the other areas listed so that the child does not attempt to make a change before he has some ability to regulate the new skill and maintain it with constancy.

Teaching representational systems of expression

These are not taught as alternative to speech but as adjuncts. Drawing will assist body image as will play. All sequential skills will be impaired so gesture and mime, if taught, will promote more skilled movement and self-awareness. Group activities may be useful and fun.

Cerebral palsy

It is easier to recognise the difficulties of children whose speech disorders arise from cerebral palsy. The impairments of motor control are apparent. But there the ease ends. The continuing treatment of such children probably makes more demands on the skill of the speech therapist than any other single group of cases. Here the lesions are in cortical areas, motor nuclei and tracts which initiate and regulate movements. As these lesions affect the immature and developing brain they will bring about selective and generalized difficulties which will become more or less dominant as the child grows. Together with the motor problems there will be sensory impairments which will further impede control. The child therefore has profound difficulty in motor activation and processing in all aspects of speech production and also in making alternative representations through visual and motor systems.

Because the brain has been prevented from developing to the mature state in which it can organise skilled movements, those that are present will be characteristic of early and basic brain function. They will operate to save and maintain life and will be reflex in character. It will not be possible for the therapist to develop, at first, any of the skilled and selective movements necessary for speech until these early reflex patterns have been brought under conscious control.

History of the management of cerebral palsy during the last 30 years makes interesting reading. It shows two strongly contrasted themes. The first, shown earlier in the personal testimony of Carlson (1941) and contained within the recent philosophy of Peto (Cotton, 1965) is that the handicapped child must struggle to achieve goals set by normal society. The attainment of these goals, walking, self-help, speech, dominates the child's development. A contrasting philosophy is offered by the developmentalists and outstandingly by Bobath. They hold that the cost to the child of attaining such goals may be harmful interference with his overall development and the acquisition of skills in a progressive, developmental manner. If he manages to walk before he has gained adequate control of balance he will not only walk abnormally, but he will never achieve adequate balance or be able to right himself with ease.

If these contrasting views are related to speech we see that on the one hand a child may be stimulated to speak in a way that allows him to express something of himself as a person and to convey needs, but he will not be easy to understand because he has not acquired sufficiently selective movements for the production of sounds. The developmental approach insists on movement through pre-speech skills and will not encourage articulate speech until the underlying prosodic features can be controlled and selective oral movement attained. Within these two philosophies lie considerable differences in tactics. The means by which movements are initiated differ in the Bobath technique to those of, e.g. Dolman and Delacato, as does the amount of sensory input to the child.

The rivalry between schools of thought on cerebral palsy management has had very unfortunate consequences in some respects; most unhappily the distress and sometimes exploitation caused to parents. But it is the opinion of the author that a strong philosophy engendering treatment methods and attitudes is extremely important in a team working with sufferers from this condition (or more properly any of the conditions comprised within the name). The team must be united and work together closely and this means common aims and understanding. The speech therapist must not only understand but actively support the work of the physiotherapist who should be the team leader. The paediatric neurologist will command the diagnostic field and take responsibility for major medical decisions but the treatment sequence of movement skills should be directed by the developmental physiotherapist. The speech therapist works with her and gains from her, adding her knowledge of speech movements to the team. She is vigilant in monitoring the child's language growth and ensuring that all other matters affecting this (for example, the state of his hearing) are properly seen to. She must also contribute her faith and enthusiasm to a team which needs to support itself emotionally so that it may support the children and parents who rely upon it.

The specific goals of speech therapy must be·seen in relation to the goals of the team, but the same heading can be used as for previous cases.

Training foci:

Teaching relaxation and control of posture

This becomes a constant tenet. The child has a damaged nervous system interfering with movement and its regulation. He therefore has no normal automatic basis for control and must be given all possible help in achieving some kind of homeostasis. For the spastic child, extreme muscular tonicity is the key disability and some reduction of this tone by relaxation and placement techniques is the key therapy. In cases of athetosis, the child suffers from shifts of tone and therefore needs to experience a point of homeostasis from which a controlled movement can be made.

Training movement

Training patterns of movement

These develop from the major focus and are the basis on which skills are built. They should therefore precede training imitation; teaching sound production and training auditory discriminating and judgement.

This should accompany all movements for speech so that the auditory/motor link is developed.

Teaching sequential skills

Some cerebral palsied children, particularly the athetoid group, have difficulty in perceiving the sequential nature of speech. Emphasis may therefore need to be placed upon careful listening and language training in the syntactic as well as the phonological area.

Developing vocabulary

All children with limitations set by nature upon their experience should be given extra help in language building through active extension of vocabulary. New words should be introduced, explained if necessary, and re-inforced by parents and therapists.

Teaching representational systems of expression

Alternatives to speech may have to be considered by the team even with very young children. The choice of system will depend on the extent of the child's overall physical involvement and therefore the methods open to him.

Attention training has not been listed as a primary focus because it is built into the techniques of physical management which are employed. For example a child may be required to take up and hold a posture. His attention is trained as part of this activity rather than as a precursor. If, however, any child (again possibly one from the athetoid group) has outstanding trouble in this area, attention training may become a specific focus.

We may see from the discussion around therapy techniques for specifically handicapped children, that it is difficult to deal with the level at which their main problems fall without having recourse to higher levels. There is obviously and necessarily a relationship between memory and symbolic understanding and between symbolic formulation and motor activation. Children with damaged and developing brains cannot and should not be ranged along one dimension of deficit and its interaction with higher and lower function ignored. As we move on to consider those higher levels in relation to the special communication problems with which their pathology is associated, we must assume that children who have these special problems have other difficulties also. Here the higher function deficit may subsume the lower. Children with severe intellectual impairment may also have difficulty in motor planning or in speech perception. Children with pure aphasia will not be able to make use of the skills of imitation and production in a way that develops their communicative competence.

Mental retardation

This global condition accounts for the main difficulty in acquiring language after hearing loss has been discounted. As the aetiology of mental retardation comprises genetic, biochemical, traumatic and infectious conditions acting upon the immature brain, it will be seen that other pathologies are likely to occur simultaneously. In some cases there are definite syndromes of which mental retardation is the outstanding disability. In other cases, damage to the foetus at a certain period, i.e. within the first trimester, can also affect those special organs of speech and hearing which are not yet complete. Students confronted with severe cases of mental retardation must therefore be vigilant in searching for other handicaps and must go back to their textbooks of genetics and anatomy to find the possible companions of the main impairment.

A distinction may be made between those severely retarded children whose condition arises from pathology and those where there is generally poor inheritance and endowment. In the last group we see poor representation of high level skills, including language, with slow and less sophisticated development and use. With the first group we see very severe constraints indeed imposed upon the learning of any skill because of basic deficiency in brain tissue and function. Individual speech therapists have always been drawn to such children and the literature gives insightful and moving testimony of the efforts on both sides to establish communication. Now these efforts are supported and extended by the very considerable techniques of experimental psychology and special education. A notable breakthrough was achieved in the 1960s when behaviour modification techniques were expounded. Since then the skills of task analysis and programme planning have given structure to the work with severely subnormal children which has resulted in steady gains.

Work with parents of young mentally handicapped children which shows the parent not only how to assist his child's learning but how to enjoy doing so is just as important (Jeffree and McConkey, 1976). Speech therapists are learning to construct their programmes on similar lines, carefully recording and monitoring change so that parents can contribute fully and a real partnership be achieved (Warner, 1980).

Sadly many profoundly retarded children spend their lives in institutions where individual stimulation and the unique and loving relationship to maintain it are lacking. Although the speech therapist may preach the need for individual language stimulation, circumstances simply do not allow for its promotion. The job of the speech therapist with the profoundly mentally handicapped person of any age must be to help those who care for him to understand the means by which he can be helped to communicate (Byers Brown, 1966; Report of the National Development Group, 1977). The aims of communication training must be seen in relation to the child's developmental status and prognosis. At a level where independence is not a realistic aim, communication of needs is important to reduce dependency and ease the burden on hard-pressed parents and parent substitutes. At this level the therapeutic techniques will be the same as those employed with the severely cerebral palsied child, i.e. sound production and movement control. Concentration will be on the pre-speech skills and these will be extended so far as is possible into communication training.

If the developmental prognosis suggests that the child will achieve a state to which speech is appropriate, the therapist will take a more active role in training the skill. She will always do so within a framework of general language stimulation as this intellectual development is the one which is primarily affected in severe mental retardation.

The thrust of therapy must be to achieve a breakthrough into the higher levels of symbolic function. If this is not possible activity becomes built up at the pre-symbolic stage with empty chatter, echolalia and perseverative utterance, random and disorganised play and stereotyped activity.

Attention training

This is best carried out on developmental lines as suggested by Cooper, Moodley and Reynell, (1978). Many workers prefer a strictly programmed behaviour modification approach and this can be very successful. The author's personal bias is against it because of the likelihood that the child has a contribution to make which could be masked by too strictly structured an approach. The choice is for the individual therapist, but if a strict behaviour modification technique is employed the person who is to use it must be rigorously trained so that she is consistent in her rewards.

Teaching representational systems of expression

This should be carried out to assist cognitive training and the development of basic concepts as well as to provide communicative channels. Play is the outstanding activity for the child and different levels of play should be taught and reinforced by the therapist. The aim is to get to the stage where the child realises that certain things can represent others. At this point it is meaningful to introduce words. In some cases non-verbal systems may be developed as alternatives to speech.

Developing vocabulary

Words must be used to interest the child and to prompt him to respond. Vocabulary building with these children never really stops or starts. It is a constant therapeutic process because the child lacks the matrix of language into which new words can be drawn. Because of this lack, vocabulary development must be part of meaningful language behaviour; taught in a context there its meaning is clear and always used in sentences or phrases which will allow comprehension to grow at the same time. If this is not the case vocabulary learning will be item learning only (see Chapter 4).

Training imitation

Training listening

Both these skills will need attention but their timing must depend on the child's talents or deficiencies. If he is a good imitator he must be rewarded for listening so that he does not rely upon empty imitation but gets the material into his memory store. If he is a good listener but not very productive he should be trained in imitation of words so that he can gain experience of production and build up memory for motor patterns.

Teaching sequential skills

The present view is that all brain damaged people may have difficulty in this area and should therefore be helped to understand the meaning and significance of sequential behaviour. Certainly the mentally retarded child has considerable difficulty in closure, or the final detail which completes the activity. This is likely to be part of general memory impairment in some children. It can also be seen as a breakdown between short and long term memory. When working in this area the speech therapist may gain considerable help from the experimental psychologist as well as his clinical and educational colleagues with whom she will have been steadily associated.

Teaching sound production

Many mentally retarded children have severe and persistent problems of the speech-sound system. These must be scrutinised. They may be part of an organisational or planning deficiency or a memory deficit. They can be manifested in the lack of closure already referred to and described by Renfrew as 'open syllable' (1966), or they may be the result of movement difficulties. If movement is the problem it should become a focus of attention, but the movement and the sound should be taught together by attention to phonetic placement. This must be done slowly and be strongly reinforced. It must then be generalised as soon as possible to the phonological system to avoid simple item learning and spasmodic appearance in speech. Equal care must be taken to avoid perseveration by teaching one sound at a time and keeping its context very clear.

With this work we are in a very classic field of speech therapy skill and one that is well represented in the literature (Berry and Eisenson, 1956; Van Riper and Irwin, 1958). Research has consistently shown the higher than average amount of articulatory deviation in the mentally handicapped population (Bangs, 1942; Matthews, 1971). We are now concerned with the exact nature of these difficulties and find that they may be

1. Immature and persisting variants which do not impede intelligibility in young children
2. Severe phonological constraints which may be patterns of immaturity rather than deviation but which are sufficiently limiting to prevent intelligible speech
3. Deviations from conventional production associated with motor or structural deficits which might be compensated for by a more able child.

The speech therapist will gear her therapy according to the need.

An analogy may be seen with the speech of the deaf so it is worth repeating the point made in that section. The presence of one over-riding handicap does not preclude minor and individual difficulties which can combine with it to produce specific speech disorders. With both these groups teachers and therapists wish to promote the highest level of language rather than becoming too soon obsessed with details of production. But if a child is not easily intelligible, or is giving an unfortunate impression of ineptness, he should be treated for his production difficulty.

Aphasia

This is still considered to be a specific and high level impairment arising from agenesis or injury to the speech centres in the temporal and frontal lobes of the brain and their associative tracts. Such children are profoundly impaired in symbolic acquisition and outstandingly in the comprehension and use of verbal symbols. The child may be able to respond to sound and to produce it but will not be able to use it at a level where it represents the object or activity. This must be deemed a cognitive rather than a linguistic deficit.

Skilled psychological testing will show that the cognitive deficit is not generalised to all areas of learning but is rooted in language disability. Such skilled testing is essential if the child is to be educated as it will give a basis for planning education. The speech therapist's outstanding responsibility in the first instance is to help to establish the child's strengths and weaknesses by preparing him for psychological testing and sharing her insights with the psychologist and audiologist who, together with herself, constitute the investigating team. The paediatric neurologist may be able to give information as to the nature of the lesion and the state of the nervous system which will guide the team in its investigations and of course the converse will equally well apply.

To those who have worked with severely aphasic children, the distinction between them and the children who show auditory and motor processing difficulties giving rise to language disorders is not simply one of degree but one of kind. Aphasia may however still be viewed as a subgroup of this language disordered category (for a recent discussion of cognitive functioning and language disorder see Benton, 1978). Once more the speech therapist moves from the medical diagnostic team into the education team. The teaching of symbolic representations that can be used as a basis for language is a paramount and continuing need. The educational team will decide what modality will be most productive in the light of the child's psychological profile.

Training focus:

A Representational system of expression

This must be lead up to by cognitive training, matching and classification; association of symbol and object, symbol and event. The concern is to help the child understand the nature of visual and auditory representations so programmes built upon normal developmental lines are unlikely to be profitable. They will simply not yield the structured information that the child needs. Neither is it wise to spend too much time trying to find a system that the people around him can easily share. As has been stated, there are some conditions in which society has to accommodate to the person. The representations selected, drawings, models, Premack, Bliss or individually inspired must be chosen so that the child can make some sense out of his environment. When this can be shown to be happening, extension or even switching to more commonly used systems may be tried.

Speech is outstandingly preferable to any other form of communication and must be tried again and again by techniques of:

Auditory discrimination and judgement

Imitation

Sound production

once the child has learned to appreciate that the communicative behaviour of other people has some meaning.

Autism

This condition is relevant to discussion of cognitive impairment and language deficit. The work of Rutter (1968 et sequor) has helpfully dominated much of this area for speech therapists. They see their contribution as aimed at children whose autistic features arise from language impairment though some therapists are also attracted to children whose impairment is more pervasive. At the time of writing we are led in this field by the psychologists and have not made a large individual contribution of our own. Students should first be trained to observe the child's behaviour in an attempt to assess whether the autistic features are appearing because too high a level of function is being demanded. Many of the children referred to the speech therapist with the diagnosis of 'autism' are mentally retarded children whose limitations have not been recognised and who therefore take refuge in bizarre behaviour. Good developmental assessment should sort out the diagnostic picture. The child's behaviour will show a marked accommodation towards normal, if infantile, relationships when he is approached at an appropriate developmental level.

The differential distinction between aphasia and autism as a primary factor is extremely difficult even for an experienced clinician and may best arise from diagnostic therapy over time. Control of behaviour must be achieved if any improvement is to take place in comprehension. So the initial stages will be:

Training foci:

Behaviour modification under the guidance of the psychologist
Attention training, associated with the above
Imitation training, associated with the above.

If the condition then suggests a strong component of language impairment the speech therapist may proceed as in cases of language disorder. She is likely to have to make continual use of behaviour modification techniques to prevent relapse and affirm appropriate associations.

If the disorder is seen as one of profound emotional disturbance, the speech therapist has no more to offer than any other professional who can create and maintain some kind of relationship with the child. His future must be seen as one requiring special educational placement. If she wishes to continue to work with the child she must do so realistically, making her position clear and not blaming either herself or the child if miracles are not achieved (for further discussion see Reeds and Wing, 1976).

In the descriptions just given of the ways in which the speech therapist works with children whose communicative disabilities are related to pathology, the different foci of therapy have been suggested. But the general points made in Chapter 2 must also be remembered: 'to give support, guidance and counsel; the attributes that mark a caring profession', also 'to promote language use and teach language structure'. To give support guidance and counsel to children and their parents means giving time. The child's programme should never be so tightly timed and structured that the immediate worry is ignored or the underlying anxiety or despair allowed to fester. The importance of creating the right conditions for therapy has been indicated in Chapter 4 and it is extreme when the patients have severe and chronic disabilities.

The general directive regarding language must also be brought into practical management. In normally developing children or those with speech delays of a non-pathological nature, the extension of language is first through speech and later through reading. The child hears a variety of language forms used to him and as a consequence of his developing nervous system he is able to make use of them. Subsequently he will be able to cope with a more formal acquaintance with language structure in reading. A child with a damaged nervous system is first prevented from understanding and generating speech and may also be unable to learn to read. He will therefore be dependent upon specialised input, at least until he has grasped the basic linguistic relationships. The response of a child to specially selected input may be very slow and he may only learn what he has been taught but this must not be assumed. Very careful monitoring must take place to find out whether child is moving in a different manner and at a different rate to that expected.

A very useful tool for monitoring language growth at these early stages is the LARSP, offered by Crystal and colleagues in 1976 and fastened upon by clinicians with considerable gratitude. It gives a framework for recording syntax, which shows where the child is developmentally, the structures he possesses and the number of times he uses them. It also gives strong guidelines for developing particular structures and building up syntax in a systematic and useful way. It can therefore offer a unifying element to the speech therapist working with language impairment from different aetiologies.

Another unifying element is suggested by Bloom and Lahey (1978). They designate the characteristics of content, form and use as typifying language skills and suggest that normal children use language in accordance with these dictates. Thus the breakdown of language may also be seen as a breakdown of one of these characteristics. The characteristics cut across causal boundaries and are thus to the taste of those who, very reasonably, find aetiological classifications unsatisfactory as a basis for therapy. But Bloom and Lahey also point out that clinical categories do exist and should be studied. Their work is one of the few that tries to give a generalised theory and yet indicate specific areas and specific techniques for remedy. The British speech therapist is used to having to make such an amalgam for herself. The recent development of such linguistic tools as the LARSP is extremely helpful in bringing theory to the point where it suggests treatment possibilities. Mention of these tools therefore seems the proper way to conclude a chapter which has been mainly occupied by medical and educational matters and the contribution of these teams to language remediation. It reminds us that the speech therapist applies to any one case the measures that are appropriate and her ability to bring together procedures taught by several disciplines will be the distinctive feature in her success.

8

Delays and disorders in developing speech — (2)

CONDITIONS WHERE THERE IS NO DEMONSTRABLE UNDERLYING PATHOLOGY

In the previous chapter we considered some procedures which could be followed with conspicuously handicapped children. They are transferable from one clinical population to another but the amount of time spent on each, the way in which it is introduced and controlled will be specifically related to the handicapped child's need. We find that many of the same procedures can be used with children who have failed to deduce or to generate the features of a conventional language system simply from interaction with the environment though they appear capable of doing so and their environment appears to be capable of helping them. We also see that methods of investigation and treatment suggested for these children will be applicable to the population previously described.

It is almost certainly naive to draw too strong a distinction between pathological and non-pathological bases for speech disorders. Many of the conditions for which we cannot account may ultimately prove to have some abnormal biochemical element. We talk of pathology because it gives us some idea of the constraints upon language learning. If no pathology is demonstrable we have to examine the speech pattern extremely carefully to determine what has prevented steady growth. This is not the only area of examination but it is a point of departure for the speech therapist and the point where she can make her individual contribution.

Infants acquiring speech have to integrate many skills derived from acoustic, perceptual and motor bases. There may be considerable disproportion in the maturation of the cortical areas subserving language. There are also differences in the speed in which linguistic elements become consolidated, and there are, of course, discrepancies between the spoken language of the child and that of the adults who surround him. All these discrepancies give opportunities for linguistic mishap but most children manage to negotiate vulnerable periods without breakdown or distress. If they do break down it is likely to be because of a combination of unpropitious factors rather than one sole incident. A child who is slow to acquire phonological features may progress without strain if his family gives him plenty of support without excessive pressure and if his temperament is such that he can accept some frustration and imperfection. However, if a child combines poor phonological perception with a strong drive towards self-assertion and expressivity and a highly verbal and stimulating family, he may create a mismatch between his syntax and phonology which will render him unintelligible. A child of similar temperament with poor verbal planning ability may run himself into stammering. On the other hand, a child with naturally low speech endowment and poor motor skills may gain so much from happy verbal exchange with his parents that his confidence leads him quietly along to linguistic adequacy.

Many textbooks give useful outlines of development progression in language learning. The following sequence, taken from Menyuk (1978) is particularly helpful in indicating possible breakdown points

The developmental sequence associated with normal speech

0–12 months	The infant is sensitive to both segmental and supra-segmental differences in the speech signal and makes communicative interaction with his environment
12 months +	Shows ability to produce speech signals with express intention and to essay statements about objects and events
18 months +	Reveals ability to express relations between objects and events in the environment
24 months +	Child begins to produce utterances in accordance with specific rules of the language of his environment.

Few parents are so linguistically sophisticated that they will note the slow progress in discrimination and response in the first year of life so long as the child responds in some way to speech and is alert. Even if the child is under-responsive, the precise stages which are delayed may not cause anxiety. The parent is looking for large signs or real, discernible milestones and so, on the whole, is the professional. For a milestone to be late, many small subskills may have been deficient or delayed. The child may therefore need more consolidation and support at the early stage of speech development because he is having difficulty with its systematic acquisition.

When milestones are achieved the need for such support may seem to lessen. So, when the first few words are uttered, even though late, their appearance can cancel out the early delay and make people think that all is well. In some cases it may be so but in others the child may be unfortunate in his other experiences and this strikes at the shaky language foundation.

The following case history offers some support for these observations and also shows clinical management which was deemed helpful. The child was first discussed by the author in 1970 and was one of these followed up for several years as part of a small research project (1974). His case was one of those presented in summary in a paper for the British Journal of Disorders of Communication (1976) when he was designated Child No. 2. He will be referred to here as Secundus.

Case summary: Secundus, the second of two children and the only son, was referred for help at the age of 3 years by the educational psychologist because of 'lack of verbal communication and disturbed behaviour'. His parents gave a history of several episodes of ear infection with high temperature during the first 2 years of life for which the child was suddenly hospitalised. He also suffered from continuous constipation which was suspected to be of psychological origin but which was subsequently resolved medically. He was a very poor sleeper and his nocturnal restlessness robbed his parents of their sleep also. At the time of first meeting all three members of the family were tense, tired and anxious.

Audiological examination showed no abnormality and normal hearing. Early psychological evaluation showed good non-verbal intelligence and excellent comprehension. Both these factors were supported when a full psychological assessment was carried out at 4 years 8 months.

The failure of expressive language was the outstanding developmental deficit, all other skills being normal. Early babbling had been tuneful and copious but no articulate speech had followed. It was considered that this was a case of speech arrest, the cause not known but associated with emotional adjustment difficulties to which the sudden hospitalizations had contributed. Another strong contributory emotion was that experienced by Secundus upon the sudden death of a much loved grandfather when the child was barely 2 years of age. The family was offered parent guidance and speech therapy, both being considered essential and mutually helpful. Parent guidance was carried out by the speech therapist with the psychologist and family doctor acting by crisis intervention.

At the start of therapy Secundus used the word 'no' but otherwise relied upon nasalised vowels with appropriate intonation for: question, assent, doubt and vehement denial.

Therapy consisted of shared play with the therapist responding by simple, dynamic and affectionate speech to the child's vocalizations and expanding anything that appeared to be a sentence type utterance. This lead to increased vocalisation by Secundus which showed good grasp of prosodic features. He also started experimenting with words. Following this experimental stage there was steady growth of syntax and it was then possible to note the slower emergence of phonological features.

Characteristic utterances. 3 years 8 months: ə̃ ə̃ (don't know.)

4 years 8 months: ˈmãɪ gɔgɪ ɪŋ
                      (mine's got a doggie in)

5 years 6 months: ˈãɪ gɔ dɪfən çɔːç ə gaːç
                      (I've got different sorts of cars.)

6 years 4 months: ˈaɪ gɔ ə mæ ɪ ɪə dəʊ
                      ˈnəʊ wɔ æpn tu ɪm nãʊ
                      (I've got a man in here and I don't know what's happened to him now.)

Secundus did not receive constant individual therapy during this time, the focus being shifted to other skills and situations as appropriate. For example, a period of normal nursery placement was advocated to help social adjustment; a brief placement in a language class was given to provide further language support. The utterances are listed as above to show the slow growth in phonology.

We can now look again at the very early stages of the normal developmental sequence of Secundus. In his case the outstanding lag occurs in the second year of life. Having shown some early sensitivity to the speech signal (as suggested by the well substantiated reports on early babbling and alertness to speech) and having started some communicative interaction with his environment, the child failed to produce consistent speech signals and essay statements. Subsequent stages were severely delayed. Secundus when first seen was using speech behaviour characteristic of the early second year of life with verbal comprehension about 2 years in advance of this. The slow growth of phonology showed persisting constraints upon this rule governed behaviour so that the child was using the phonological pattern of a 2 year old when he had a chronological age of 5 and a syntactical age of around 3 years 6 months. As the syntax had reached a level containing all the major elements and might be expected to develop subsequently in a normal manner, the phonological constraints were deemed to need attention.

The timing of therapeutic intervention is essential to its success. If corrective tactics are applied too early they may inhibit natural growth. If applied too late they will be impeded by the emotions that have become focussed on the disability, or they may be impeded because of the strong habit factor then operating. Judgements about intervention are influenced by the child's attitude and feelings and by the therapist's estimate of his position. In this case the development of well formed sentences was not being accompanied by expansion of the phonetic inventory (see Ingram, 1976). Study of the growth rate and stages of syntax and phonology would prompt a therapist to decide in favour of phonological intervention. Study of this particular child, his temperament and needs also prompted this activity. There could be children where the decision is complicated by a lack of congruence between linguistic timing and temperamental timing and these must be considered individually by the therapist, but her considerations will have more solidity if she has something of the framework of ideas which has been described.

Secundus's vulnerability was compounded by his chequered emotional development and it will be seen that a major area of linguistic delay was in the early laying down of normal phonological patterns. Whether he would have had any difficulty in speech perception and discrimination at a very early age independent of his emotional difficulties remains speculative. It can only be recorded that he did experience sudden separation and distress during his infant years and was then 'unable to make any relevant response that would resolve the discrepancy or bring the child closer to his parents' (Musser, Conger and Cagan, 1974).

With such a child the therapist tackles direct speech correction only very slowly and when confidence between the child and herself has been established over a long period of time. In this case the direct work took the form of practising phonemic contrasts in imitative and competitive games; recording each other in the process; writing and reading to each other nonsense and then sense words containing the contrasts and then using them in picture form in further competitive games (e.g. pelmanism or picking up twos). The ability to engage in competitive activities which the child wins but only just is also a required skill in speech therapy. Once more, the techniques are simple but if properly based in knowledge of the theory and knowledge of the child they may be relied upon to work.

A different course was pursued in the case of another boy, also presented as part of the 1974 study. He is listed No. 8 in the British Journal paper and will be referred to here as Octavius.

Case summary: Octavius, at that time an only child, was sent to the audiology clinic at 2 years 7 months by the medical officer for delay in speech onset. A co-operative test of hearing (appropriate for the child's age) did not reveal significant hearing impairment. There was also response to high and low frequency sound at minimal intensity when the results were checked by distraction testing.

Octavius responded to simple instructions and attempted to communicate with the therapist by sounds with strong intonation. Sounds were mainly vowels but simple consonant/vowel combinations were used in naming [ba-ba] (baby), [tʌ] (truck). He could be stimulated to imitate simple words but showed difficulty beyond one syllable. Some jargon type utterances were noted. Octavius's communicative behaviour seemed to be at around the 18 month level, i.e. he could signal some differences in his own utterance and could comprehend simple utterances by people other than his parents. He was attempting to essay statements and express relations between objects albeit in a rather primitive fashion. He related well and maintained good interaction with his environment.

It was considered that Octavius had the basic attributes for speech to develop and that his affectionate and insightful mother would be the best person to help him. As neither parent was highly verbal, some suggestions were made to them as to how they might talk more to their son. The suggestions were specific, as such suggestions need to be. They concentrated on play-time, bed-time and week-end outings. Demonstrations were given and discussed as to the ways in which the boy's speech attempts should be expanded. There was no local speech therapy and the family had to travel some distance to attend for guidance sessions. Because of illness and one or two other domestic difficulties the sessions were less frequent than planned.

Re-assessment at 3 years 5 months showed only very slow growth of syntax, with much higher than average proportion of nouns to other words. Simple two word combinations were the longest units essayed spontaneously though with stimulation these could be developed into longer, though still simple narrative, e.g. 'car crash' expanded to 'man car crash dead'. Octavius's strategy seemed to be one of stringing nouns together rather than developing any phrase or clause structure and there was a conspicuous absence of verbs.

Attempts at sentence imitation showed severely reduced utterances of a telegrammatic kind, e.g. 'boat on the water' was reduced to [bəu wɔ:wə].

It was now apparent that the child was not experiencing a simple developmental delay in acquisition but a marked difficulty in combining words into longer units. The quality of the speech showed that the phonology was correspondingly delayed in that even the simple words uttered were not spoken with good consonant/vowel detail and final consonants were omitted. The position needed re-appraisal first from the diagnostic angle and second from the therapeutic.

If his position is checked against the developmental sequence we see that the child is essentially still at the level of skills appropriate to the very start of the third year of life. If checked against the LARSP scale his utterances fall into stages 1, 2 and 3. (This procedure was not carried out at the time because the LARSP had not been published but as the corpus of language had been retained it has been possible to look at it subsequently). We see that when length is attained it is at the cost of the natural variety of grammatical forms which would be normal. The therapist, seeing a pattern developing which is slow, laborious and not indicative of linguistic ability has a responsibility towards the child to look again.

Hearing re-assessment showed conductive loss of 45/50 across the range. Fluid in the middle ear was indicated by impedance measurements and Octavius was referred to the ear, nose and throat department. He was treated first medically and then surgically, the latter by tonsil and adenoidectomy and myringotomy. Normal hearing was not shown until following these procedures when Octavius was 4 years 6 months.

It was tempting to hold the fluctuating levels of hearing responsible for the speech delay. The possible effects of such loss have already been pointed out in Chapter 3. Morphological features would not have been consistently audible to the child and consonants of low acoustic energy would also have been lost. But the original late development of sentences prior to the loss and the particular language strategies employed by Octavius did not support this hypothesis to the therapist's satisfaction. He was therefore referred to the psychologist for a fuller investigation of his verbal and non-verbal skills. Results showed non-verbal intelligence to be normal, and his verbal comprehension to be 3 years 5 months for his chronological age of 3 years 8 months. His expressive language was estimated at 2 years 4 months. The Reynell Scales were employed for both language measures. The psychologist considered Octavius to have a significant problem in expressive language and suggested that a full psychological re-assessment be carried out before school placement was decided, that is at about 4 years 6 months.

It was now considered that the evidence of language disorder was sufficient to change the focus of therapy from simple expansion and re-inforcement to structured teaching. The general speech stimulation given might have been reckoned to help Octavius compensate for his hearing loss and his verbal comprehension level did not suggest severe difficulty in speech input. The most likely hypothesis was verbal planning difficulty affecting all sound sequences but particularly word order. If this planning difficulty was present the hearing loss would have compounded its effects. Therapy was now concentrated on teaching sentence forms in statement and question and on devising play in which these could be practised. This work was then handed over to the mother and the therapist concentrated on sound imitation to develop phonology. Later the therapist took up the syntax work to give the child more alternatives and the mother carried on with drills to establish clear production.

This case reminds us of the need to alternate our interest between the child's developmental skills and language sequence and his underlying attributes. We have to note the pattern of speech and its rate of acquisition, both of which are exceedingly significant, and then check to see whether the factors underpinning these skills are present. We therefore examine a variety of sub-skills which are built into the acquisition process.

Sub-skills underlying normal development of speech
    Auditory acuity
    Auditory discrimination
    Vocalisation
    Oral sensation
    Oral movements   Feedback
    Babbling – physiological: Demonstrating motor/sensory integrity
    Babbling – linguistic: Demonstrating auditory/motor coupling
    Intonation – auditory: vocal feed back
    Linguistic recognition: auditory skill + cognitive maturation
    Prosody – as above + regulation of output
    Words – as above + association and memory
    Word combinations – combination of all above processes
The final product, clearly articulated, flowing speech which uses grammatical forms to convey meaning, has to be nurtured by these sub-skills. We do not as yet know the extent to which each has to

be present but if the desired product fails to emerge it is sensible to see which sub-skills are lacking. We may then be able to trace strains of difficulty to which we can direct therapy or areas of vulnerability for which compensation is required.

Careful investigation of all skills and sub-skills is necessary when the presenting symptom is of failure to acquire fluency. Much careful work has gone into describing the difference between stammering (stuttering) and the normal non-fluency of the developing child (Williams, 1971). Stammering is likely to take place where any discrepancy exists between thought and word, content and execution, desire to speak and fear of speaking. Whether it actually does so will depend upon temperament, anxiety, pressure and other unquantifiable commodities which influence the speaker. But the speech therapist confronted by a young child whose parents are worried about his stammering must certainly assure herself that he does have the verbal forms, the content and the use to allow fluent speech to develop. If there are inadequacies of vocabulary: auditory memory, sequential skills, planning and motor processing, she will try to buttress these while reducing the anxiety on the part of the parents and the child. If no area of inadequacy is found the cause of the stammering must be sought in the relationships between the child and his family or in any other emotional and environmental circumstances which are preventing the confident exchange between family members.

Case history: A very typical case for the speech therapist is that of Magnus, a large, well-grown child of 3 years 10 months who is considered by his parents and doctor to be slow in learning to speak. The developmental history shows late motor milestones, notably walking. Handedness is undecided, eye hand co-ordination is poor and the child is noticeably clumsy. Although late in starting to speak he had progressed steadily and is now talking continuously using simple sentences. He shows immature articulation which the parents describe as being 'poor' or 'babyish'. Recently they have become concerned because of the amount of hesitation and repetition they had noticed in his speech and the increase of aggression in his play. They attribute both activities to the effect on Magnus's life of his younger brother now aged 10 months.

Case history: Another case is that of Benjamin, third son of a lively, able family with professional and highly verbal parents. Both older brothers are extremely intelligent and the whole family is highly competitive. Benjamin started to speak rather late compared with his brothers but not so late as to cause concern. He always showed a good level of vocabulary but his production of words was not always clear and he still, at the age of 4 years 1 month has occasional substitutes of [y] for [l] and habitually replaces [r] by [l] and [θ] by [f]. His parents are concerned about the increased amount of stammering, or repetition with tension shown in his speech. He is also bed-wetting more frequently than he did. They associate this with the birth of their first daughter now 3 months of age.

Both these cases show the child at a stage where it is easier for him to get worse rather than better. He has been particularised, brought for investigation and shown to be a focus of family anxiety. The speech therapist pays heed to the presenting symptom, that of non-fluency or in Benjamin's case, stammering and uses it as a signal for investigation. The two basic questions are:

Does a problem exist?

If a problem exists what is its nature? (for further discussion of these questions see Muma, 1978).

These two questions are strongly related and in order to answer them the therapist has to consider both the parents' points of view and the child's. She will probably proceed in the following way:

1. Informal session with the child in the presence of his mother. Attractive play materials will be provided and the therapist will talk naturally with the child to find out more about the ease with which he communicates. This session will be recorded as are subsequent sessions until a good corpus of speech has been obtained. The recording will then be analysed by the therapist with regard to syntax, phonology and amount of non-fluency or stammered utterances. The therapist will then make her personal decision as to whether she considers the child to have a speech problem.

2. Proceeding concurrently the therapist will have an informal talk with the child's parents during which time she may find out how anxious they are and what is their opinion of their child's ability. She will use the case history as a means of checking what has given rise to the anxiety. She will make some decision as to whether the parents are justified in believing the child to have a problem and she will then put her two decisions together and look at both of them. Some such conclusions as these may arise.

Magnus: All aspects of spoken language delayed but developing. Syntax expanding rapidly; phonology unstable. Very good interaction and no obvious speech inhibition. Incidences of non-fluency confined to situations in which several ideas are being expressed.

No marked aggression in play with people or farm animals. Bossy but reasonable in play involving therapist. Not unduly egocentric; likes to dominate but will take turns. Comments on his performance to mother and asks for her approbation but only rarely.

Magnus's parents: Concerned about child's immediate future. 'Will he speak clearly by the time he goes to school?' Also his long term future. 'Does the speech difficulty mean that he is not very intelligent and if so what sort of school will he need?' Also concerned with immediate management. 'What should we do when he hits his sister – is rude to his mother – is disobedient – and should we correct his speech?'

The parents show no real difference in attitude towards their son's difficulties. They have obviously talked about their fears to each other and the visit to the speech clinic is the result.

The combined effect of all these factors makes it likely that the therapist will answer the two basic questions in the following way:

Does a problem exist? – The grounds for a problem exist but the problem should not develop

What is the nature of the problem? – The imbalance at present manifest between the child's speech standard and motor skills and his temperament and ideas.

This leads to the next question: what should be done about it? The following procedures are indicated:

1. The parents should be given a good account of the child's language skills and their significance explained. The relationship between delayed motor control and speech delay should be discussed.

2. If the parents wish, a psychological assessment should be arranged at a later date so that they are given a clear picture of the child's assets and likely educational future. If the speech therapist has gained an impression of normal intelligence and this is substantiated by the child's play and demeanour she should not hesitate to point it out.

3. The state of Magnus's speech should be used as a baseline for continuing evaluation and the therapist should see him at regular intervals to assess growth. The length of the intervals will depend on how the parents feel after the first discussion and how the child progresses.

4. Magnus should be given plenty of alternative outlets for his energy, such as those provided by play group or nursery. His father should be asked to help improve his physical co-ordination by outdoor sports and also by building and constructional games.

5. Non-fluency should be seen as a temporary inadequacy by the parents who should encourage the child to sort out his ideas in

speech by appropriate questions and expansions but without correction. They should continue to talk naturally to him but take every opportunity to tell him stories, anecdotes and give full verbal explanations when asked so that the child may hear pleasant and purposeful language. They should not be afraid to speak firmly or discipline him when he is being wilful or to restrain him when his roughness could hurt other people.

Benjamin: Compliant but restless during play. Tended to give minimal answers to comments until the play became interesting, then talked readily with the therapist. Stammering was noticeable in approximately one out of every three utterances and in all long utterances. It was frequently accompanied by increased fidgeting. Audible intake of breath could be heard on the tape recording preceding some statements.

Benjamin used good sentence structure and assessment showed high verbal comprehension and vocabulary levels, but he sometimes failed to respond to speech and frequently replied 'I don't know'. When taken through the Edinburgh Articulation Test he said 'I can't say it' to the stimulus pictures 'umbrella' 'yellow' and 'feather'. He looked anxiously at his mother several times but did not ask for her approbation.

Benjamin's parents: The father was very concerned about the child's speech and also his bed-wetting. The mother, while concerned, believed Benjamin to be an intelligent child and thought he would learn to speak properly. She also thought that the child was very sensitive and needed to be treated more patiently by his father. However, she was very worried about possible jealousy of the baby sister as a cause for the boy's stammering and bed-wetting and confessed to feeling guilty lest she was responsible because of mis-management.

The parents seemed to be looking at the child from somewhat different viewpoints. The father was mostly concerned about the child's inadequacy and the mother about her own. The father therefore corrected the child and tried to get him to speak in a different manner and the mother did not. The father had frequently commented on Benjamin's stammering but had not really discussed the matter with his wife until agreeing to accompany her to the clinic.

The combined effect of all these factors makes the following resolution likely.

Does a problem exist? – yes

What is the nature of the problem? – the child's anxiety about his speech and his parents' inability to help him or each other.

So: Benjamin should be enrolled in a programme of speech therapy designed to improve his fluency and his confidence. This could take the form of listening and modelling, with time given to repetition of modelled phrases by the child in order to improve feedback. Sentences should be simple and clear so that no burden is placed on the child's memory. Recordings should be made of Benjamin's good utterances and these played back to him for further repetition. Discrimination training should be given in preparation for stabilising the sound [l] and discriminating between that sound and [r]. Production should not be started with [r] or [ɵ] and it should be explained to the child that these are sounds that a lot of older boys have trouble with. A promise to teach them at a future date should be made (and kept).

These procedures should be interspersed with creative activities like drawing, modelling and puppetry during which natural talking can be encouraged. A small group of children with like difficulties would be a suitable setting for both forms of treatment once confidence had been established and a relationship formed with the therapist.

Concurrently with help for the child help must also be offered to the parents. This should best take the form of discussion with contributions from both sides. It is desirable that both parents adopt the same attitude towards the child's speech and his father should be advised not to correct him. He should also try to relieve his wife's feelings of guilt over time spent with the baby and give Benjamin more of his time to make up for this. If so that time would be best spent in non-competitive activities such a reading to the boy or watching television together. As Benjamin grows more confident his relationship with his father can be allowed to develop more robustly and more competitive activities encouraged.

The children, Magnus and Benjamin are used as illustrations of the way the therapist proceeds. There are many other possibilities implicit and many other conclusions possible.

All the children presented to illustrate points so far have had parents who are genuinely anxious about their welfare. The management shown by these parents was not necessarily helpful in overcoming speech difficulty but that management was nevertheless prompted by real affection and concern. Unfortunately there are very many cases where the parents are not at all concerned about their child's speech or may even be responsible for his communication difficulties. It is well established that speech is a learned skill, requiring interaction between the developing child and an adult who cares for him. If this interaction cannot be established or maintained during the formative years, the child will not speak normally even though he may have the physical and mental potential to do so. A recent and tragically extreme demonstration of the effect on a child of severe deprivation may be found in 'Genie' (Curtiss, 1977). Other, less extreme effects can be seen in young children left all day in institutions with very few staff to tend and love them and in those who spend a high proportion of their waking hours in the care of child minders, themselves preoccupied by their own domestic tasks and lacking the tie of devotion which allows a mother to keep her infant underfoot and still communicate continually in a way that he can understand and respond to.

We should make a distinction between the young child who is considered to be linguistically deprived because there is little communication in the home and the child who fails to acquire the skills which other members of his family have developed because of particular circumstances or attitudes which militate against him. The child who is deprived or 'disadvantaged' because of his social class and economic circumstances is the target of a great deal of interest by sociologists, psychologists and linguists. The speech therapist cannot fail to have her own interest stirred nor to perceive the connection between deprivation and communicative disability, but the broad remit of the linguistically disadvantaged is not hers. Her skills are needed for the individual who is more penalised than his peers by such circumstances because of other factors which are particular to him. While it is entirely proper that students of speech therapy should be acquainted with the literature on social deprivation and linguistic disadvantage, they should focus their interest on those children who are conspicuous even within this environment.

There are many children who lack the care which promotes communication. They may be considered in the following manner:
1. Children who are being neglected by adults
2. Children who are being punished by adults
3. Children who are being mishandled by adults.
Once more the point must be made that individual children make individual demands. Some infants seem to emerge from the womb more demanding and more vociferous than their siblings and do not respond to the same treatment. Others are naturally less affected by adult behaviour because of some built in placidity or self sufficiency. There are children who are crushed by a comment which their brothers will oppose spiritedly or ignore. It may nevertheless be helpful to illustrate these categories with individual

cases although the children cited may have been individually inclined towards language delay.

Case history: Una aged 4 years 3 months, was brought for speech therapy by her foster mother. The little girl and her brother of 2 years had been found alone in the streets late at night and the family had subsequently been investigated by the social services. The social worker appointed to the case had found Una's mother incapable of attending to the children because of drink. The father was away from home for periods of time because he was employed as a maintenance worker on an oil rig. There was no lack of affection in the home but the mother had become increasingly depressed and was unable to face the demands of running a home for her children without her husband's support. The house was neglected and the children were left for long periods of time without supervision. The Social Service Department had started to help Una's mother deal with her own problems but pending her ability to do this the children had been taken into care. Psychological examination of both children showed the boy to be only just below norm in language as well as motor development but the girl to be 18 months below the verbal norm for her age. In addition, Una showed considerable ambivalence towards her brother, sometimes emulating his play and infantile utterance and other times being fiercely aggressive towards him. It seemed likely that this ambivalence had arisen from the mother's declared preference for the male child, though she did not believe herself to show this.

Speech assessment confirmed the linguistic level estimated by the psychologist and found no real discrepancies between phonological and syntactical development. It was therefore decided that the child would benefit most from a programme of language nourishment and reinforcement, and that this should be associated with play. This programme was carried out by the foster mother in order to help the child establish a firm relationship with her and because of her good opportunities for re-inforcement. As Una might return to her mother at some future date the therapist saw her at least once a month with the object of keeping an essential element of stability in the language programme.

Focus of therapy: Una had reached the stage of simple two word combinations with the majority of her utterances falling into the two-element sentence or stage 2 (Crystal et al, 1976). Her younger brother was at approximately the same stage or slightly below. There are obvious reinforcing factors which could keep Una's speech at this level. These are as follows:

Lack of the necessary language input on which to model sentences

Lack of loving reinforcement to stimulate experiment

Lack of incentive to essay more mature utterances and the further delaying factor of identification with the younger child who appears to be more lovable.

Therapy must therefore aim to move the child along by providing the necessary model:

Giving all possible positive reinforcement

Suggesting ways in which incentives and rewards can be built into communicative activities

Helping to build up the little girl's sense of self regard and identity.

Simple play activities can again be used and in Una's case they should be built round situations in which she has some control and where she can use her speech to manipulate others. Doll play would be very suitable.

Therapist: 'Where's baby?'

Una: 'Baby bed'

Therapist: 'Wake baby up and tell her its time for breakfast'

Una: 'Baby, baby. Wake up baby'

Therapist: 'She's very sleepy this morning isn't she'

Una: 'Baby tired. Naughty baby.'

Therapist: 'Oh, perhaps she needs some more sleep. Shall we leave her in bed'?

Una: 'No. Naughty baby. Get up'

Therapist: 'You get baby up then if she's just being lazy'.

The therapist is obviously not attempting to give the child structured and selected input but rather to help her convey ideas through speech. The use of simple play allows the child to work out her feelings and reveal her attitudes at the same time as practising speech. It has the advantage of being easily demonstrated to others and so being reinforced with the minimum of difficulty. These play methods are used continually by speech therapists for children with delayed speech. The cause may be deafness, mental retardation or deprivation but the basic idea of expansion round role play is useful in each case. The difference would lie in the amount of supportive information given, the clarity of response demanded and the speed of growth expected. In Una's case growth should be speedily accelerated. The therapist uses her other main contribution, that of regular assessment, to oversee and safeguard this growth.

Case history: Joshua aged 3 years and 2 months was brought to the speech therapy department for assessment because of lack of speech. He had failed several tests of hearing, the most recent at 2 years 6 months when it was suggested that acuity was probably within normal limits judging by objective audiometry but that the boy was not able to co-operate sufficiently to give a clear picture by co-operative testing. He showed responses to high frequency and low frequency sounds at minimal intensities but these could not be repeated. There was a suggestion that the child was withdrawing and failing to relate to people. The question of possible language disorder was raised.

Joshua is the child of West Indian parents living in very poor accommodation. His mother is at home with the child and a younger son and at the time of her visit was 5 months pregnant. Joshua's father did not attend the clinic with his wife and had never accompanied her on any of her clinic visits. Information from the health visitor suggested that Joshua's mother was completely tied to the home and had no relatives or friends to visit her. There has been complaint from neighbours about the children's crying and the noise of adult shouting and quarrelling.

Joshua showed only very fleeting attention to the therapist and ran about the room until restrained. He responded to physical restraint by wriggling and crying but did not speak. He went in immediate pursuit of any toy on which his eye lighted and showed protest and distress when prevent from putting small toys under his jersey. He failed to understand such statements as 'you can play with it when you sit down'.

Such a presenting picture could herald a condition of autism, mental retardation, hearing loss or aphasia. A period of observation and discussion with Joshua's mother and the health visitor however revealed the following. The parents had not adjusted happily to life in this country having come over here immediately after their marriage. Joshua's father had been in steady employment but did not like his work in public transport and complained of discrimination against him by employers and workmates. He resented time spent with his children and was intolerant of Joshua who had been born very soon after his mother's arrival in Britain. He did not actively ill-treat the boy but tended to shout at him and to use threats. Joshua was required to keep quiet when his father was sleeping during the day following night shift. Housing conditions were very cramped and it was difficult for the boy to play without disturbing his father.

Joshua's mother also displayed resentment towards the child because of his demands. He had been a fretful and tiring baby and she was at present unable to toilet train him. She attributed much of her isolation to her necessary early occupation with Joshua as a baby and saw him as establishing a pattern of demand in which she had been trapped ever since. She admitted that when she felt very depressed she tended to vent her feelings on Joshua and that she felt most fond of him when he was asleep. Moreover, she was now irritated by his lack of speech and associated this with her failure to toilet train him.

This picture of unhappy and resentful parents making the child the scapegoat for their circumstances and feelings, is, of course, one with which social services are extremely familiar. The onus is upon that department to assist the family and in particular to provide support for the mother. The obvious suggestion is to put Joshua into a day nursery to give his parents relief and the child additional care. The speech therapist must be prepared to assist by seeing the child for individual therapy in order to awaken his interest in verbal communication. While his situation seems very similar to that of Una there are important differences. Una had been given attention during the pre-linguistic stages of speech development and had absorbed and could produce the basic elements of the language structure. She had not been penalised for attracting attention and she had been given affection by both parents though not in a stable manner. Joshua had lacked a warm response from his mother to his early sound play and this had cancelled out his interest in vocalising as a means of attracting attention. Neither had he received much pleasure from the speech of others. The whole 'trick of language' had eluded him because its significance had not been pleasurably demonstrated. In order to encourage any speech growth there would have to be very strong and consistent reward for vocal activity and listening.

Focus of therapy: Joshua has not yet laid down the information and responses appropriate to the first year of life in that there is a lack of communicative interaction with his environment. An immediate attempt must be made to establish this. Joshua's parents should not only receive support from social services but guidance from the speech therapist so that any attempt made by other people to establish this interaction does not break down because of negative reinforcement at home. If Joshua is placed in a day nursery one person must be allowed to give him individual time so that the link of sound and reinforcement is forged and listening may begin.

Such cases as these are often very disappointing unless approached realistically because a team effort can easily fall apart from sheer practical circumstances (see Chapter 3). Unless some attempt is made to work with Joshua he will almost certainly become less and less amenable to interaction. Until some attempt has been made to interest the child in language and to reward him for communicative effort no predictions can be made about his linguistic future and no fair assessment of his abilities can be carried out.

Case history: Regina, aged 2 years 10 months, was brought to the speech therapy department for help following audiological assessment. She was able to carry out a pure tone hearing test which showed a good level of cognitive development and the test revealed normal acuity. However, the audiologist commented on her unusual speech. This consisted of glottal sounds produced with great rapidity and emphasis with all syllables being correctly stressed in two and three word utterances but no articulation of consonants and vowels. Thus, in response to 'here's your chair' Regina said [a a i e] (that's Daddy's chair).

She showed very good comprehension for speech and a high level of representational play. Physical examination revealed no abnormality of the oral structures and Regina's mother reported that she ate normally and had never had chewing and swallowing difficulties.

Regina, an only child of middle class parents was accompanied to the clinic by both her parents and they seemed to be interested in her welfare and concerned about her lack of 'proper' speech. Further investigation however revealed the following situation. Regina's parents were in the process of seeking a divorce and had been living apart for the past nine months. Each had found another partner and was proposing to re-marry when their divorce was finalised. Regina lived with her mother but saw her father every day. She appeared happy and showed no signs of disturbance but each parent now blamed the other for the child's lack of speech. According to her mother, early infant babbling had been normal and comprehension had always seemed good. Early words 'mama' 'no' were normally uttered and there was no anxiety aroused by anything in Regina's speech behaviour until about 6 months ago. At that time Regina started to use sounds to attract attention rather than attempting to shape words. Her father, according to the mother, had laughed at this and encouraged the child to be 'silly'.

Now Regina was persisting in the same kind of utterance but her father was annoyed by it.

According to Regina's father, the child was spoilt by her mother and no consistent discipline imposed by her. The child therefore 'did what she liked' and her mother did not oppose her. Regina's father believed that the child's speech should have been checked by her mother instead of 'letting it become a habit'. He was opposing his wife's plea for custody on the grounds that his daughter was suffering because of her mother's neglect. Regina's mother was pleading that the father should not be given custody or even frequent access because he 'interfered' with the routine which Regina needed and because he was not prepared to give his daughter consistent and regular attention.

Once more the case presented is a familiar one in the records of social and legislative prescription. Here are two parents whose child is being used by each to exemplify the faults of the other. Any short-coming on the child's part or any deviation from the norm would be identified by each parent as the adverse effect of the other's management. It was obviously important to establish how much the child had been damaged by these attitudes. Assessment and observation in fact showed a competent and intelligent small child who was easily able to manipulate her adult relatives. Her early speech attempts had first been received with interest, then with amused interest and then with concerned interest. All in all, Regina had little impetus to change her way of speaking and considerable interest in maintaining it. As an unusual pattern it attracted attention and gave the child plenty of opportunity to enjoy adult response. Without presenting as a disturbed or neurotic little girl, Regina showed good aptitude for adult exploitation.

In a case like this the speech therapist has to foresee that any sustained interest on her part could reinforce the idea that the child has a real speech dificulty. She must therefore decide whether the danger to the child of failure to make use of a systematic phonology is greater than the danger of being particularised as someone with a speech problem. Fortunately time is on the therapist's side. The child is young and she has good inner language. She is able to generate sounds and control some aspects of their production. If the therapist wishes to make a change at this point she may do it:

1. By persuading both parents to adopt a different attitude. This must mean not responding to Regina's abnormal speech pattern. This is a dangerous path since it requires harmonious and con-

certed action by two people who at present see each other as enemies.

2. By establishing some interaction with the child which will demonstrate the advantages of normal utterance.

If the therapist elects to follow the second course the following action is appropriate.

Focus of therapy: Imitation. Regina must be tempted to see that it is interesting and fun to explore sounds and verbal play. The therapist will therefore use 'echo' games, role play and puppetry to encourage systematic exploration of phonemes. When she is satisfied that Regina can produce sounds in all classes and comprehend language at her age level she may leave the integration to other circumstances to promote. If the child reveals competence and practises activities at all speech levels (sound play, discrimination, word imitation, directing others through use of single words) and simultaneously shows good understanding of linguistic content she will certainly put these things together when required. It then behoves first the parents, then the nursery or school to make appropriate demands so that Regina's performance may improve.

It is less easy to refer Regina's state back to our developmental sequence than it was with the other two children. She could be seen as having taken time out from an ascending path to wander fitfully elsewhere. She has left the track at around the 2 year stage where 'the child begins to produce utterances in accordance with specific rules of the language of his environment'. As the basic stages have been safely established there is plenty of under-pinning for the rule governed behaviour. The therapist tests out the child's ability to appreciate a rule, to discriminate between utterances and then to produce the essential element that it needs. The choice of whether or not to abide by the rules must be the same as that made by any other person, namely the one of conformity against idiosynchrasy. Self-interest is likely to determine the outcome.

The disorders of speech described and illustrated in this chapter are those which used to occupy the 'functional' category of a classification system. As has been suggested, this distinction between 'functional' and 'organic' may be much too crude to allow for the intricate interaction that is taking place in a developing child who fails to conform to average expectancy. But it must be pointed out that many of the problems presented are those of personality and could therefore be seen as the proper remit of the psychotherapist or child guidance officer. As always the question is one of emphasis. Where the speech appears as a kernel difficulty even if not causative, there are strong grounds for seeking speech therapy opinion. If the emotional difficulties are pervasive and do not seem to be focused upon linguistic inadequacy, the psychotherapist or psychologist is the person to take charge. If there is any doubt, the matter must be resolved by proper and co-operative discussion so that the child, already at risk because of adult inconsistencies and jealousies is not further threatened or deprived.

9

Persisting speech disorders

We must now consider those children whose speech disorders persist beyond the age where maturation can be expected to play a large part in remedy. It may be seen from the discussion of causal and perpetuating factors in Chapters 7 and 8 that there will be children with such severe neurological and structural impairments basic to their speech handicaps that normal utterance is never a realistic possibility. For these children we must seek the best accommodation possible and must co-operate in finding special educational placement if their communication handicaps make it impossible for them to benefit by normal schooling.

The report of the Committee of Enquiry into the Education of Handicapped Children and Young People, (Warnock, 1978) emphasised the need for a continuum of care for all children found to have special educational needs. This care should take them through the first stages of assessment and parent guidance into school and subsequently follow their careers in both special and normal education. It should also provide for adjustment into the adult world of employment and social intercourse after leaving school.

The contribution of the speech therapist to early assessment has already been discussed. Grady, writing on language and the pre-school child in 1973 stated that such assessments must indicate that spoken language is

1. In the process of change
2. Being acquired slowly but non-deviantly
3. Being acquired slowly and deviantly.

Prescription for specific speech therapy or nursery placement and guidance would be indicated by these assessment results. Even if appropriate action is carried out at this time there will still be children entering school with spoken language of the kind indicated by Grady's categories. We may find children whose language is still evolving towards the norm but who have the basic structure well established. The children may need some additional support or reinforcement but it is likely that they will continue to make progress without specialist intervention. Children whose speech is being acquired slowly albeit non-deviantly may not have a system adequate to bear the load of further cognitive and linguistic skills without continued specialist help; those who are acquiring language slowly and deviantly will certainly require specific and continuing treatment.

Children may also appear at school showing language delay who have not received an early assessment. Their speech difficulties need to be investigated to determine their nature. So, however good the pre-school service, the need for screening procedures at school age cannot be obviated.

A comprehensive screening programme to identify speech disorders is by no means easy to devise. Screening for hearing loss works on present/absent criteria with the child signalling his response to sounds of different frequency. In spite of the abuses of the procedure and the difficulties often encountered in carrying it out, it does identify the child with severe hearing loss and, if well administered may pick up the mild problems also. Speech tests are much more difficult because you are testing not for the presence or absence of a specific response but for the presence or absence of many features none of which may be significant in itself. A child who started to speak late may be showing articulatory immaturities which are much less significant than the poor prosody and word finding difficulty of the child with a real language disorder. But the latter could pass an assessment that was entirely directed towards articulation of standard consonants and vowels.

Articulation of speech sounds is only one of the processes involved in normal language acquisition. Siegel and Broen (1976) consider the components of language most often implicated in speech and language disorder to be:
1. Articulation and mastery of the phonological system
2. Understanding and use of grammatical structure
3. Understanding and use of vocabulary
4. The functional or interpersonal use of language.
Screening tests administered by other than speech therapists are mostly concerned with intelligibility which involves element 1. and possibly element 2. There is no way of testing out the last two factors without individual assessment. Moreover even the first two factors may escape a superficial examiner since the sounds and words may be available to the child in limited context but his difficulty lies in processing and producing them systematically. Thus children with comprehension and language learning difficulties

which may be highly pervasive and penalising in their effects can elude examination. If the child has limited but clear utterance his comprehension and language use will not be tested further and these may be very vulnerable areas indeed (for an example of such of child see Byers Brown and Beveridge, 1979). We must therefore cling to the concepts of early referral for delayed speakers and a continuum of care if we are to give proper service. But speech therapists will also continue to experiment with screening procedures which will identify both the kind of speech which is likely to be a problem in itself and the speech that is likely to be connected with general or specific language impairment and thus affect other language forms.

Disorders revealed in the articulation and mastery of the phonological system are those with which the speech therapist is traditionally connected and where she has built up a high degree of expertise. Articulation testing has occupied much of the literature on speech assessment.

The history of such testing is well recorded (Irwin, 1972; Powers, 1971). It has moved from testing single sounds and consonants in initial medial and final positions to testing them in all possible phonemic contexts. It seeks to probe a child's phonetic inventory and to record this in a way that will act as a baseline and a measure for progress in therapy. A very popular articulatory test in this country is the Edinburgh Articulation Test which allows a pattern of normality, deviation or immaturity to be seen and therefore has some diagnostic and prognostic value. Students are well trained to use such tests and generally derive confidence from the clear cut procedure and the information yielded.

A very important function of any measure of articulation is the extent to which it can predict whether the difficulty is likely to persist or whether it may resolve itself without specialist aid. Renfrew writing on this point (1973) emphasised the need to save the 'overstretched speech therapy service' for those children who would not improve without much help and therefore the need to find some way of identifying those who might. This comment was partly prompted by the recently received results of the 7 year old follow-up of the 1958 cohort (Butler, Peckham and Sheridan, 1973) mounted by the National Children's Bureau. This study gave information on the prevalence and persistence of speech disorders in the 7 year old population. It revealed that 10 to 13 per cent of the children had some degree of impairment (Peckham, 1973). It was considered by speech therapists that this might be a very conservative estimate as the survey was carried out by doctors and teachers, the former using ratings of 'fully intelligible'; 'almost all words intelligible'; 'many words unintelligible' or 'nearly all words unintelligible', and the latter reporting children whose speech was 'somewhat' or 'certainly' difficult to understand.

The group identified by doctors as having almost all words unintelligible and by teachers as being 'certainly' difficult to understand was subjected to further study. Records of 286 children were thus scrutinised and a group of 215 with 'marked speech defects' emerged. These were exclusive of hearing impairment or stammering. The group was far from being homogenous and included children with dysarthria and all forms of language disorder.

The 215 children emerging from the NCB study 'came as a whole from lower income homes, and the children were later members of large families. They had been later in walking and talking, were more clumsy, had more visual defects and demonstrated more emotional disturbance than the controls. Their performance in reading, number work, copying-design and draw-a-man test was below average' (Sheridan, 1973). We therefore have a strong association between speech disorder and education and a suggested one between speech disorder and neurological dysfunction. Such associations have been made many times among smaller groups of children but there is value in having the position restated as the result of a national survey. It is not the purpose of such a survey to demonstrate the exact nature of the link between the three conditions. Its results are valuable in drawing the attention of those in charge of services to the relationships and thereby to future needs, but for the speech therapist and the teacher who have to apply remedy, the lack of information on the exact nature of the link between speech disorder, educational failure and neurological impairment is frustrating. Once again we are confronted by a group of uniquely handicapped individuals who may, or may not have a great deal in common. The more they prove to have in common, the more likely they are to be able to receive appropriate education help. Prescription for an individual child in an educational authority with limited means is likely to remain Procrustean and speech therapists are only too aware of the results of such prescription. It is therefore worth reminding others of what these difficulties mean in terms of human suffering.

Case history: Luke was referred for assessment and advice at the age of 8 years 9 months. At that time his speech was frequently unintelligible and he showed general language disorder with a severe reading problem. Basic to his speech difficulty appeared to be the inability to monitor his utterance and to maintain a consistent standard. He was able to control simple elements of utterance but as they became longer in construction and demanded more complex phonetic patterning his performance deteriorated. At this point both intelligibility and fluency broke down.

Medical history: Luke was a premature child, normally delivered, with a birth weight of 3 pounds 7 ounces. He was in an oxygen tent for about 4 weeks following birth. He had subsequently thrived and suffered no severe illnesses.

Development history: All motor skills were somewhat delayed. Luke sat up unsupported at between 9 and 10 months and walked alone at 2 years. Speech was more severely delayed than any other skill. No words were recognisable until 4 years 9 months at which age he started speech therapy.

Social history: Luke is the third and youngest son in a family of four children. Both parents are alive and well and both are concerned about Luke's welfare though his mother takes the more active part in seeking help for him. He has become very isolated at school and in the small rural community where he lives. His mother, teacher and therapist believe this to be due to his communication difficulties as the boy is both responsive and affectionate.

Progress: Educational and speech progress are almost at a standstill hence the referral. Speech therapy had earlier concentrated on developing a communicative system and developing representational skills. This had proved helpful but there was now need for a much more intensive programme of remedial and linguistic help which the present local authority was unable to provide.

Hearing assessment: No impairment; a pure tone audiogram revealed normal acuity. Luke tried hard to be helpful, and cooperated fully but attentional difficulties were apparent. There was also instability of posture with sudden small movements indicating shifts of muscle tone. The fluctuations revealed were outside those of normal range. The medical audiologist commented that the boy had poor fixational control and that his nervous system did not appear capable of handling a normal load.

Psychological assessment revealed abilities within average limits on both verbal and non-verbal intelligence testing. A reliable WISC profile was obtained in which the detailed results showed a scatter of abilities including 9 years 6 months on verbal comprehension and 6 years 6 months on digit span and 6 years 10 months on picture arrangement.

The psychologist commented on the results of testing digit span as revealing particular difficulty in sequencing auditory imput. The revealed deficiency affected matching of auditory and visual sequences and proved to be of significance in relation to Luke's extreme reading problems. These problems impeded reading to the extent that the boy was limited to a very few phonically simple words of two or three letters. While knowing the sounds of some letters he was virtually unable to synthesise the sounds of any phonically regular two or three letter words. Any attempt to synthesise sounds impaired recall.

A remedial programme was immediately suggested and implemented to incorporate these findings and my own, which are here quoted.

'Luke uses speech as his usual means of communication. He volunteers statements and responds readily to questions and comments. However, it is apparent that he still has a severe language disorder. He shows word finding difficulties and is unable to monitor his speech effectively in units longer than short words. In longer and more complex statements he degenerates into unintelligibility although he is obviously attempting to keep the conventional semantic and syntax structure.

Luke's voice is toneless, lacking in rhythm and variety of pitch and he has difficulty in regulating his speed. His articulation contains immaturities, and he also distorts and elides sounds but the overriding characteristic is blurring of sound structure associated with lack of synchrony of movement. When asked to repeat sentences he made a very good attempt reaching 12 and more words. But he was unable to maintain clarity of utterance while trying to recall and reproduce verbal content.

Luke was able to imitate single consonants and consonant/vowel combinations but could not alternate them at speed. He showed discrimination difficulty within the fricative consonant group and could neither imitate them accurately nor reproduce his own repetitions at speed. He was unable to reproduce intonation or melodic cadencies and could not sing in tune.'

The speech assessment had preceded the psychological one and had indeed led to a request for the latter with the recommendation 'that all aspects of language and learning be fully evaluated in order to suggest a programme for the further development of reading, writing and verbal expression. Particular attention needs to be paid to sequencing skills in view of the kind of difficulties Luke is experiencing in speech.'

We have here the case of a child where there has been no wilful neglect, whose early difficulties were recognised and who was given as much help as the local authority considered it could afford to provide. We have also a very unhappy boy who cannot speak so that other people can understand him, cannot read, cannot write and whose co-ordination difficulties, although slight, prevent him enjoying mechanical skills or competitive games. He has the very good assets of a devoted and articulate mother and good intelligence. He also has the support of his local speech therapist and teacher who have struggled to find further help for him.

Luke's nervous system must have sustained some damage that prevented development at the normal rate. There was consequently no gradual move towards the organised plasticity which allows skills to be developed and integrated. One could postulate that a state of disorganised plasticity had been followed by rigidity and inhibition. Instead of language being nourished by a normal matrix of neuropsychological sub-skills it had been built upon certain accomplishments only. These accomplishments were the higher cognitive attributes which ensured symbolic representations and the lower level ability to generate the individual sounds of speech, but there had been no gradual coming together of perceptual and productive skills and no integration of movement and representation.

Children with these individual difficulties who live in sparsely populated areas pose considerable management problems. Short of sending the child away to a special school at a very early age or moving the whole family to another area, there is unlikely to be any real solution. Speech therapists are often asked whether solutions of this kind should be contemplated. The question demands very thorough and objective discussion. In this case the family had been unable to move and the consensus of opinion was not to send the child away. Although the decision was made in everyone's interests when Luke was a young child, it was one that was being seriously questioned at the age when he was referred to us. By that time it was apparent that there were no facilities locally which could unite to meet the boy's needs and that the best that could be hoped for was a combination of remedial class placement and speech therapy. It was not possible or indeed desirable that such a combination should try to support the boy throughout his school career. Unfortunately it was by now rather late to enter his name for one of the very few schools for children with severe language learning difficulties. This was nevertheless immediately done and pending action on this front, the suggested programme for the development of language skills was worked out and implemented. This programme had in fact to be relied upon for a considerable period of time before a place at the residential school was available. Once admitted

Luke made excellent progress but was obviously still going to emerge as a handicapped youth with 'special educational needs'. The next phase, that of finding some training for him upon leaving his special school, is now under active consideration.

We will now review Luke's case to see what would have been the ideal support and teaching system for him had the opportunity been available.

Handicaps	Needs and provision	Remedial team
Slow development of early motor skills	Physiotherapy to improve eye-hand co-ordination, balance, spatial perception and body image	Physiotherapist and parents
Slow response to speech	Listening and sound discrimination to be stimulated by presentation of interesting sounds and words as child learns to maintain regard and concentrate his gaze on person or object	Parents guided by speech therapist
Little vocalising or utterance	Mother to be shown how to stimulate babble and sound play by physical handling and appropriate sound response to develop tune and melody	Mother guided by speech therapist
Difficulty in co-ordinating movements in play	Gradual presentation of toys and tasks to assist body stability, independent hand movement, fine finger control; also larger activities of throwing, catching, hopping, kicking, etc.	Father guided by physiotherapist
Poor auditory sequencing	Increase listening span by presenting words of different length, e.g. 'jam' and 'marmalade.' Then improve listening for length and detail, e.g. 'Marmaduke the cat is the colour of marmalade.' Encourage appropriate intonation and prosody	Speech therapist supported by parents

Handicaps	Needs and provision	Remedial team
Poor concentration	Increase time spent on all the above activities and take them into less protected and more taxing situations	Family
Delayed and abnormal utterance	Teach sound contrasts; encourage imitation of sounds and their use in words; teach and then expand two-word utterances; teach and encourage normal prosody	Speech therapist
Inability to cope with normal infant class	Small language unit	
Slow and deviant language development	Syntax building programme; if phonology does not expand sufficiently give additional training in feature perception and imitation	Teacher and speech therapist Speech therapist
Diminishing	Phase back into normal infants school for part of the day; review progress	Psychologist, speech therapist, teacher

A concerted programme of this kind would have given the child the best start. The continuum of care would then operate to ensure that he maintained his place in normal school without too much strain. The team may now be lead by the medical officer who would keep in touch with the child and his family to oversee his physical and psychological health. The psychologist would re-assess the child at intervals or on request to see whether further remedial teaching was necessary and what kind. The speech therapist would give periods of concentrated work at developmentally and socially demanding times to help the boy adjust to these demands. She would also be prepared for a policy of 'crisis intervention' should there be regression in speech or development of stammering.

The actual situation being rather different, we must now consider the programme actually suggested for Luke and see how it should be geared to give most benefit. We should first consider the programme rationale in relation to the boy's difficulties.

Speech (present position)	Deficits
Pitch control	Unable to vary pitch in continuous speech nor of short units, e.g. vowel glides
Volume control	Good increase and decrease of volume on vowel glides and simple words but not when coping with articulatory detail or normal sentence structure.
Auditory discrimination	Some ability between single phonemes; very poor in running speech. Unable to distinguish between three repetitions of 'l' and the sequence 'l, m, n'
Auditory sequencing	See above. Unable to repeat the word 'lemonade' accurately after several practises of the consonant sequence 'lmn'. Managed after several trials to get as far as 'lemona' Quite unable then to say 'melon' but perseverated on 'emon'
Phonology and syntax	Basic structures and relationships present but very variable standard of performance
Fluency	Poor rhythm and occasional stammering

We see many areas of vulnerability for which Luke has tried to compensate by memorising content. His good score for verbal comprehension shows his strengths here. This is supported by his sentence repetition skill. There is outstanding difficulty in re-processing sounds for different word sequences. This skill is basic to articulate speech and to reading and is therefore doubly handicapping. There is evidence of impaired feedback in both proprioceptive and auditory processes.

Approach to therapy
In view of the need for a stable structure, a sustained attempt must be made to improve auditory control. A hierarchy must be established so that he can practice monitoring:

The word
The phrase
The simple sentence
The compound and complex sentence.

Word structure must at first be simple, not containing too many sound contrasts and then become more demanding.

Although a hierarchy of skills is required for graded practice the approach should not be a developmental one. Luke is long past the stage where he can be helped to graft linguistic units into a matrix of prosody. He does not have the prosodic underpinning to make this reasonable. If he is taken back to a level at which he can achieve smooth synthesis and sequential ordering it will be a long way below the level of articulate speech. Neither is his condition such that he can compensate directly for the weakness of one modality by the strength of another. His best attempt to do this is in the example already given when he uses content to assist his memory for structure. Consideration was given to using this strength to develop linguistic resource and thus try to make up for speech and reading difficulties at the phonological level, but this was not deemed helpful. It would leave him too vulnerable at the level of word analysis. On the other hand too much hammering at the weak phonological area could result in failure and frustration – also in fatigue and thence depression.

It was therefore decided to teach distinctive features of sounds to the level at which they could be recognised and reproduced accurately. As soon as this basis had been laid down attention should be given to the mastery of polysyllabic words. The hierarchy of monitoring suggested above should now be used and should develop into sustained narrative and discourse. At the same time drilling on morphological changes that signal plurality and tense should take place. When, and not before, there is control over phonology and morphology in simple and carefully monitored speech, its practice may be combined with reading and phonics used in word analysis.

The psychologist and teacher built up their reading programme to strengthen visual and word recognition and to make utmost use of this until the auditory modality had been retrained. The two skills were then brought together in the matching of auditory and visual symbols, the words being said aloud as well as read silently. Finally more attention was paid to phonetic detail and strong phonic support was added to the reading scheme.

The word finding difficulty commented on at the time of referral was not made the focus of specific therapy. Word finding is associated with many kinds of language difficulty–language formulation under stress, in fatigue, in anxiety and in states of distraction. It was considered that Luke's basically good memory and interest would enable him to recall words if he was not having his attention drained off into the structural detail of speech. If he gained confidence in his ability to produce the correct sequence of sounds in words then he might be able to use some of his creative energy to finding appropriate words. Also, as his reading improved he would be able to extend his vocabulary naturally, with pleasure and without anxiety.

If we once again look at the schematic representation of language processes we may see that the main foci of therapy were directed towards strengthening the very weak links in the whole process and that this was done through reconstructing rather than constructing.

The higher level processes were used to assist in compensation as distinct from developmental therapy where the lower builds towards the higher.

Compensatory level

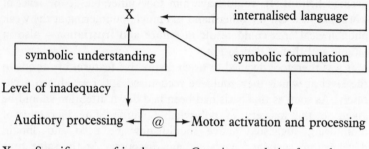

X = Specific area of inadequacy: *Conscious analysis of sounds*

@ = Major area of strength: *Memory*

☐ = Areas of strength

⟶ = Therapeutic focus

The areas of strength are isolated from the areas of weakness and cannot support them adequately. Some means of developing the links between the processes must be found.

In the earlier publication to which reference has already been made (Byers Brown and Beveridge, 1979) the author referred to questions which need to be posed about the nature of speech difficulties and educational problems:

1. Is there a continuum of language disturbance seen initially in the acquisition of spoken language and later revealed as defects in the secondary systems of reading and writing?

2. Can we assume that all children with initial disorders of spoken language must be at risk educationally?

3. Is there one underlying factor which is causal and which thereby links all language manifestations? Or are the skills all related by factors in the child's disposition, either neurological, emotional or environmental but not causally linked?

In Luke's case the evidence seems to suggest a continuum of disturbance because of the nature of his early speech problems. His educational difficulties were therefore predictable. There is also some evidence to suggest that although he had many sensory/motor problems contingent upon his damaged but developing nervous system, the factor of auditory functional impairment had strong effects on both speech and reading.

Learning disorders

The Warnock report designated four main categories of learning disorder in children. *Specific, mild, moderate and severe learning difficulties*. Each of these groups may be expected to yield children who have suffered from early language delays and may be experiencing language disorders. It is for the psychologist, speech therapist and teacher to worry out the nature of the link in the individual case. A great deal of work in the area of *learning disorders* or *learning disabilities* has come from the United States. A comprehensive attempt to look into the relationship between language and learning disabilities in children and adolescents has been made by Wiig and Semel (1976) (see also Wiig, 1976 and Lapointe, 1976). The work of Wiig and her colleagues shows the extent to which detailed testing can reveal areas of deficit and therefore offer remedy and has yet to be emulated in this country in a comprehensive way. The individual speech therapist cannot hope to get far without the help of an interested psychologist. If one such is not available she must rely on the many assessment tools which she is trained to use and which can give her information but she must be cautious about making too many educational pronouncements because of lack of knowledge of teaching methods.

A distinction must be drawn between children who are able to make sense of language but generate it irregularly and the children who suffer from *severe language disorder or aphasia*. If the latter have not been identified early there is little hope that they can be helped at school age by piecemeal intervention. They have an outstanding need for special educational methods and these must be carried out in protected environments (see Chapter 7).

The special schools and units which exist for the severely language impaired have tended to develop their own programmes based on simplified language structure. Much of the early work was dominated by the associative methods of McGinnis (1963). All teaching schemes used in such institutions need to be highly structured so that the children have their attention focused on what is basic and essential to language understanding and use. It is difficult for therapists working in non-specialised clinics to make use of these methods because they cannot control the situations in which they are taught and reinforced. It is simply no good toying with a little part of a language scheme that is meant to develop from systematic and regular exposure to concept and symbol. As Cooper and Griffiths have pointed out (1978) these types of language failure need direct and systematic language intervention in a specially designed educational setting and even then their ability to develop language skills may be very limited. It is therefore as important for teachers and therapists in this area as it is for those in cerebral palsy to attain some unifying philosophy as well as producing practical training programmes. Any severe and limiting condition makes heavy demands on the people trying to ameliorate it and each team member needs to contribute to the overall aim and to the team buoyancy.

The leader of the speech therapy service in any given area must know what kind of provision to make for her persisting population of speech-handicapped children. It is important to know how many children have difficulties which are not going to be resolved before junior school by a judicious mixture of guidance and intervention but where there are likely to be long term demands on the speech therapy service. It is always helpful to have more than one speech therapist involved with long term cases and the present structure of services is just starting to make this possible. The senior member of the team is available to her junior colleagues who may be at a loss as to what to try next or simply fearful that the child is failing to improve because of her own deficiency. There will be some children, who need to be thought about afresh; who have a new manifestation of an old problem; who have only recently considered themselves or been considered to have a problem.

Tactics and strategies must be revised and modified accordingly.

Phonological disability

The question of intelligibility is highly relevant to considerations of tactics and strategies. No therapist is happy if the child's developing speech is not allowing other people to understand him more easily. Some of the impediments to intelligibility have already been discussed. In many children with impaired central nervous system function there is likely to come a point where the final major obstacle is the lack of 'smooth triggering of successive target movements' (Dalton and Hardcastle, 1977). These children may be categorised as 'apraxic' and the thrust of therapy redirected towards improving the movement from one sound to another rather than striving to elicit a larger phonetic repertoire.

Other children who show persisting difficulties which impede intelligibility may be quite skilled in organising movements and in maintaining a system of sounds but this system differs from the speech of the child's peers and from the speech of adults who might be expected to influence him. These children appear within the category of *phonological disability*. A characteristic case history for such a child is that of William (Chapters 2, 4, 7). Development is normal except for a delay in the onset and development of expressive speech. When the speech does develop there is a greater than average discrepancy between growth of syntax and phonology which affects intelligibility. Another typical history is of early start of speech and good early motor development. The production of sounds however fails to increase at a rate commensurate with the child's communicative needs or with the complexity of the ideas he is trying to express. So the cognitive and syntactical aspects of language move far ahead of the sound system that the child developed when he was first attempting to communicate. These children do not show pathology and no cause for the abnormality is established.

This group of children is of great interest to linguists who are attracted towards them because of their deviant phonology and the absence of other problems which too often clutter up the research field. They do not present the messy picture of attentional difficulties, intellectual immaturities or motor incompetencies which get in the way of data collection. The contribution of linguists to the speech therapist's care of such children has been outstanding and indeed revolutionary (for brief history of this contribution see Grunwell, 1975). We owe to them the concept of the mismatch between linguistic systems and skills. In many children the constraints upon phonology may prevent syntax expanding into full sophistication but the major discrepancy is between the thoughts that the child can express and the sound system he uses to do so. It is this discrepancy which caused intelligibility problems. It obviously follows then that the more elaborate and abstract the statement, the less intelligible the child will be.

Phonological disabilities are likely to be well established by the age of 4 years 6 months and if so the child is not going to improve as the result of therapy which concentrates only on sub-skills. The desirability of direct linguistic intervention as soon as the limitations on growth are recognised is strongly advocated by this author. Her opinion is shared by many but by no means all of her colleagues so once more the student is urged to consider the individual circumstances before defending her partiality at the child's expense. The later the description of the deviant phonological system is made the more likely it is to be accurate in its working out of the rules, but intervention given earlier may stop the rules becoming too constricting and may therefore keep the child moving (see William, Chapter 4).

Most of the descriptions of deviant phonology offered by linguists in their studies of child language are of the speech of children of 5 years or more (Compton 1976; Connor and Stork, 1972; Grunwell, 1975 and 1980; Ingram, 1976). But Cruttenden in his discussion of such an exercise (1972) reminds us that no child's system is truly 'fixed' and that if one uses the term 'system' it is important to stress that some parts may be firmly established, other parts erratically so and yet other parts only in process of establishment. There is discussion in the literature as to whether the child with deviant phonology recognises that his own speech differs from the adult model. Examples are quoted of children failing to respond to their own version when offered by an adult but insisting on making the adult change his production to the mature version. Smith shows the recognition of contrasts by the child well before he is able to produce them and suggests that this is a normal developmental stage (1973). As such it may appear late or be perpetuated in children who show phonological restrictions. The child continues to operate on two systems, one for comprehension and one for production.

An interesting extension of this premise, which is well recognized by speech therapists is seen in the case of twin boys (Byers Brown and Beveridge 1979). These children not only distinguish between the adult system used to them by their parents and other adults but between the different systems offered by each other. (example)

Robert:	ˈdæ ə ˈdeɪn
Therapist:	Yes, its a train.
Timothy:	ˈaɪ nɔu cɪ ɪ ə ɪ ə bleɪn
Robert:	ˈnəu mi: dɪn ɪ ə ˈdi:dl
Timothy:	ɪ ˈwʌ ɔ e nu: di: ʊ aɪ ˈɪn
Therapist:	Is it a diesel or a train?
Robert:	ɪ ˈnɔ ə ˈwein ɪ ə dɪdl
Timothy:	ɪ ə dɪʊ

The fact that each child responds quickly to the content of the speech whether offered conventionally by the therapist or idiosynchratically by his twin suggests that he is not highly attentive to speech detail. This allows him to move forward intellectually in that he is not at a loss to understand nor to formulate, but it is not going to assist him in changing his own production. In order to promote change the therapist must first analyse the child's phonological system to see what features he possesses.

Timothy 4 years 3 months
Sound repertoire
In initial positions: b d m n w l r j

In medial positions: m n w l j ʔ
In final positions: mn ʔ
Rules or tendencies
Tending to omit sounds rather than substitute others
Absence of velar sounds
Absence of voice/voiceless contrast with all consonants voiced
Tendency to bilabialise clusters thus:
Try [blaɪ]
Climb [blaɪ]
String [blɪ]

Syntax only slightly delayed and *vocabulary* and *content* levels high. Consequently there is a significant mismatch between the levels of phonology and syntax with the possibility of this increasing as syntax develops to convey ideas. Open syllable is a marked feature. Timothy is not often intelligible outside his family circle but does not appear to realise that his speech forms differ from those of the adult.

Robert 4 years 3 months

Sound repertoire
In initial positions: b d m n w l j
In medial positions: b d m n w l j ʔ
In final positions: m n   l   ʔ
Rules or tendencies
Tendency for consonants to be voiced
Tendency for final consonants to be omitted
Vagaries
Occasional appearance of velar in final position
Clusters reduced in various ways:
Tree [d i]
Train [d e ɪ n / w e ɪ n]
Slipper [l ɪ ʔ ə]
Sleeping [ʊ ɪ ʔ ɪ n]
Scarecrow [l ɛ ə d ə ʊ]
Stamps [j æ m]

Syntax about a year delayed and *Vocabulary* and *Content* levels high.

In Robert's case there is a rather closer match between phonology and syntax. Although the repertoire of sounds is also very limited the phonemes are used in a more versatile and slightly more mature way. Intelligibility is somewhat higher than his brother and the phonological system appears more amenable to change.

While both boys need attention concentrated upon phonology

these findings suggest that Timothy needs to be made aware of the voice/voiceless rule; the existence of velar sounds and the significance of word endings. Robert needs assistance, through auditory discrimination and imitation to stabilise and expand his phonological system. It must be said firmly that attempting to change the phonology of lively children who are busy with their own concerns and unaware of the effect of their speech upon other people, is a very difficult task. The speech therapist owes it to the child to encourage verbal communication even though he is not readily intelligible. If she is too restrictive the child will decide that speech is difficult. This is a harmful decision and one which is very hard to reverse. If she is too permissive the child will think that his speech is acceptable and will then become perplexed and indignant as people fail to understand him. An introduction to change has been described in the case of William (Chapter 4). The therapist invokes the aid of the family and tries to get some sound shifts or some expansion of the phonetic repertoire. If successful, she may then be able to help the child incorporate the sounds into his phonological behaviour and use them to establish phonological rules. For example, William having learned to say 'dinner' will be introduced to the word 'tin'. Minimal pairs can be used for training in the rule and then activities devised to 'put the puppy's tin p(l)ate under the table'.

Anyone who has worked with a busy and imaginative small boy will know that at this point the activity can take over and the therapist find herself feeding imaginary dinosaurs out of a coca-cola bottle. But the alternative, which is to keep the child working on drills at the table and then hand him over, boisterous and frustrated to his mother with the request that she 'practise at home' is palatable to no one. Many of the variations produced by speech therapists to bridge this time gap have fallen down in their effects because of lack of control over the child's environment. They have also fallen down because the speech therapist is ambivalent about the method to be pursued. There are, after all, still a number of choices.

1. To work on syntax in as controlled a manner as possible in the hope of encouraging systematic linguistic exploration by the child which will have some spin-off into phonology
2. To build up the child's imitative and discriminatory skills and hope that he will become more facile in producing a range of sounds which may later be incorporated into a system
3. To proceed slowly on the lines of articulation therapy, exposing

the child to 'new' sounds in the hope that they may gradually be incorporated.

It will be seen in the light of previous discussion that 2. and 3. are not really viable techniques for children with phonological disabilities. They also result in criticism of results by other professions. It is not uncommon to read that a child of 6 'has been in the care of the speech therapist for 2 years but is not intelligible'. Moreover the many cases cited by linguists of the introduction of new phonological principles for children with speech disorders (see previous references) nearly all start by saying that the child, now aged 6, has been having 'conventional speech therapy' without effect. The argument is not really so simple. If a change in the child's phonological system is to be brought about at an early age the conditions must be propitious (see Chapter 4 on therapeutic environment). The same arguments does not apply in the case of an older child. While his therapeutic and domestic environment may make a very considerable difference to his progress, the therapist can deal with the child in such a way as to make the maximum use of his own abilities.

Children who are unintelligible at 7 years of age or so are likely to be frustrated and depressed, but they are also likely to want to change. They wish to be understood and to be accepted. They are used to a somewhat formal teaching day at school and will therefore be prepared to accept a working clinical session. They can be reached by verbal discussion of alternatives. They can use interesting gadgets without getting too carried away (see Fawcus, 1980).

The child Secundus, cited in Chapter 8, had different treatment at different times by the same therapist. The time for corrective work was clearly indicated by the boy himself. During a resting period following work on language interaction, Secundus's mother found him moping in his bedroom after school. Hoping to cheer him up she asked him what he wanted for his birthday. After a certain amount of listless responding the child suddenly said 'Mummy, what I really want is to talk properly'. His mother telephoned the therapist next day and she, of course, seized this God-given opportunity to start work on phonology.

Another child, brought to the speech clinic for assessment at the age of 7 failed to respond at once when asked for information. The therapist, believing him to be showing anxiety rather than ignorance or aversion said to him. 'You look as if this is going to be hard, but we are only going to talk and talking is easy'. She was rebuked for her naivety by the child's response [ɪʔ ɪbm iːbɪ ɔː miː]

(it isn't easy for me'). The therapist is, of course, given opportunity for retrieval 'No but I can show you how to change so that it will be easier and people will understand you. Let's get started'.

So the speech therapist, convinced though she may be of the importance of early intervention, charmed as she may be by the behaviour of young children, and inspired as she may be by the challenge to her creativity and ingenuity will nevertheless find the ages of direct explanation a considerable relief.

'In our language we have lots of different sounds. We make them by putting our tongue into different positions and by moving our lips and jaw. You can see some of these positions in these drawings (show diagrammatic representations). The sounds belong to different groups or families depending on where we make them and how we make them. All these sounds belong to one family because they are made with a little explosion [t, d, k, g, p, b] but they are not all the same because they are made in a different place. We can put all our sounds onto a chart so that you can see how many there are and what kind they are (suitable version of normal phonetic inventory table attractively presented using colours).

You are using this sound [g] most of the time. It is a perfectly good sound but it only belongs in some words. Let's make a list of the words it belongs in.

Now let's imitate some of the sounds on the chart. Good, you can make a lot of these sounds. What we have to do now is to work out where they go so that you can learn to use them instead of having to use [g] so much.'

The subsequent therapy programme would be based on the phonetic chart but the therapist would still have a number of interesting choices to make at different points. For example: 'You remember that we put the sound [z] on a word when we want to show there is more than one. One table, two tables, one chair, two?– Yes, chairs'

Therapist	Child (looking round the room)
One picture	Five pictures
One wall	Four walls
One pencil	A lot of pencils

Continue this for as long as possible. *Therapist*: 'Now tell me quickly all the things you can see in the room'. *Child*: 'A table and a light and some chairs (*Therapist*: 'Good') and a mat and some pictures ('good') and some toy (look of silent protest from therapist) and some toys ('good').' OR *Therapist*: We put the [z] sound on a word when we want to show there is more than one: 'Here is a picture of one animal doing something. Listen–the dog (is) playing with the ball. Now tell me about this one.'

Child: 'The dogs (are) playing with the balls'.

In other words how swiftly the child moves from a single example to a generalised rule will be determined by the child's aptitude. The example given was morphological but the same process can be illustrated phonologically.

Therapist	*Child*
Make a whispered sound using the back of your tongue	'k'
Now make a whispered sound using the front of your tongue	't'
Now make a whispered sound using your lips.	'p'

'I'm going to put those sounds in nonsense words and you've got to change them so that all the sounds use your voicebox'.

Therapist		*Child*
ee k ee	eekee	eegee
ay t ay	aytay	ayday

Continue, making child self-correct.

Therapist: following the teaching of voice/voiceless–'I'm going to give you two words that are almost the same: Coat and goat. The only difference is between the [k] made with whispering and the sound [g] made with voice. Now I'll give you a sentence to read'

Child: (reading) 'A cap is near the coal.'

Therapist: 'Fine. I'll draw it for you'–'Here's the next sentence'

Child: 'The gap is near the goal.'

Therapist: 'Good. You are the footballer so you can draw that one.'

Therapist: 'Now we will say the sentences just from looking at the pictures.'

After many repetitions

Therapist: 'Now tell me what I've drawn.'

Child: 'A cap.'

Therapist: 'Where is it?'

Child: 'Near the goal.'

Therapist: 'Who do you think it belongs to?'

(if she is lucky) *Child*: 'The goalkeeper.'

(more likely) *Child*: [tɪn ɪ piə] = I think it's Peter's

Therapist: 'Or perhaps the goalkeeper? Could we practise that?'

Speech therapy is the art of filtering complex ideas into simple procedures. It is necessary to find this simple basic level with every child and then make work increasingly interesting by skilfully applied motivation and by use of equipment. By getting the first stages of the process established with clarity the therapist allows the child to experience positive success. He will then be better able to cope with a more complex phonological exercise. The child himself can explain to his teacher what he is doing and thus maintain authority and develop control. He will also be encouraged to continue the regular practice which is absolutely essential if he is to make any progress. Adults should not deceive themselves into thinking that a swift transfer into normal speech can be achieved by a child who is just starting to rebuild his sound system (for further elucidation on this point see Fawcus, 1980). The choice of sound contrasts to train, or of new placements to require, will be made on both developmental and experimental criteria and the only dicta are that the procedures must be systematic and well supported. They should be preceded by thorough phonological analysis made from a taped recording of the child's speech during informal activity and supported by specific testing of words and phrases or constructions as indicated.

Writers at the present time are concerned to emphasise the difference between children with phonological disabilities and those with articulatory difficulties (for full review of articulatory field see Winitz, 1969). A child such as the one referred to in Chapter 3, child C, will certainly present at school age with residual articulatory difficulties. He has not had the practice to become skilled in producing accurate patterns of speech at speed. Neither has he reached the developmental stage in sound acquisition where complex sound clusters, affricates and other sophisticated phenomena are appropriate. The therapist will intervene in cases like this if the child shows distress because of inability to acquire sounds or if his rate of acquisition and improvement in skill reaches a premature plateau. She should not intervene and try to force the child along because of pressure from adults though she owes it to interested parents and doctors to give them a history of the child's speech and some guidelines as to what to expect. She must be ready to support parents who may suddenly lose confidence because of this kind of pressure and she must always be ready to reconsider in the light of new evidence.

The category of residual articulatory difficulties will have been one of those tapped by the National Child Development Study. The group of persisting speech defects must have included children with conspicuous difficulty in producing a number of sounds in a normal manner, but the group may not have included a number of children who show slight variation in manner of production affecting one or two sounds only. This group is the old one of 'simple dyslalia' as named in the early days of the College of Speech Therapists terminology (see Chapter 6). It was subjected to some scrutiny by the author in co-operation with the Manchester Speech Therapy Service lead by Mrs Brenda Kellet. The overall object of this exercise was to see what kind of speech disorders predominated among the Manchester population of 7 year olds and also to look at the diagnostic categories into which therapists placed their children. After discussion with all the therapists involved the category 'phonetic' was agreed for those children who at 7 years of age had persistent sound distortions or substitutions which could not be seen as part of an overall impairment of articulation and which did not represent part of a deviant phonological system (for helpful discussion of phonological and phonetic representation see Grunwell, 1980).

Phonetic deviations
The children identified by the Manchester therapists as having minor articulatory anomalies had been handled in a number of ways. These are worth recording because they show more of the decisions which have to be made by speech therapists. There were 17 children in all.

8 were under regular but infrequent supervision
2 were attending for therapy
1 was awaiting therapy
2 had recently been discharged
4 were listed but no determination arrived at as to how they should be handled.

The children were agreed by the investigators to show the following: Seven children had slight structural or neurological deviations from the norm. These were sufficient to interfere with speech and, in the opinion of the investigators sufficient to prevent normal production of certain sounds. These children could not therefore be expected to change their production and could never reasonably have been expected to produce the sounds normally. Their acceptability would depend on the importance of correct speech in their lives. If the need was great a more acoustically acceptable sound would have to be aimed for. Otherwise there was no point in giving them therapy.

Four children were considered to show some immaturity overall in syntax and phonology:

One had a history of conductive hearing loss
One showed some residual dyspraxia
One was socially deprived and possibly ESN (M)

One showed variability in production affecting more than one sound

together with occasional omission of syllables.

Three children showed faulty production of one sound or pair of sounds with no other abnormality. It was considered that these children were most suited of the 17 to be categorised under phonetic deviation.

Every speech therapist has a number of children known to her whose speech is not absolutely correct but which she deems to be no deterrent to the child's emotional, social or educational adjustment. The speech difficulty seems too slight to merit firm categorisation. If the errors become targets for anxiety the therapist will use her judgement as to what to do. It will be quite obvious from listening to public speakers that articulatory vagaries are no deterrant to success but, should they become so the person is entitled to help. Adults with individual speech problems of this nature are certainly well worth working with if their motivation is high.

Cases of phonetic deviation should be differentiated from those who show dental or inter-dental speech across a number of sounds. Such speech is likely to be associated with abnormal tongue action which may be difficult to change. Most of the literature on these cases comes under 'tongue thrusting' and involves orthodontists as well as speech therapists in the search for remedy (Van Thal, 1954; Ballard and Bond, 1960; Gwynne Evans, 1972).

Another condition or group of conditions best dealt with in the specialist literature is that of voice problems in children. These do not present very frequently in the speech clinic but they always have strong medical implications. Persistent or frequently occurring voice loss, pitch abnormality, lack of volume, gruffness or hoarseness should not reach the speech therapist unless the child has been seen by an otolaryngologist. If they do present without medical opinion treatment should not be given until this has been gained.

The final major class of persisting speech disorder, stammering, will be discussed in the next chapter. Its relationship to language disorder has been indicated but its manifestations are more appropriately discussed elsewhere. Those speech disorders persisting into school life which have been the main target of interest have been those which will inevitably interfere with secondary language representations unless handled by combined therapeutic and educational methods.

Failures of maintenance and homeostasis

Some of the attributes which a child needs to develop competency in language and pleasure in speech have been suggested already in these pages. The speech therapist's role in assisting him in his development has also been indicated, but it is impossible to describe all the experiences and attitudes which accrue to establish an adult as a confident speaker, at ease in the world of verbal communication. Students of speech therapy are required to study developmental and social psychology and to be acquainted with psychiatry in order that they can have some idea of the influences on individuals and the possible personality deficiencies which makes those influences overpowering. Students are themselves sensitive and growing people and if encouraged to consider their own experience and become objective about it will develop insight into other people's behaviour. But we must all remember that we share a very small part of time with our patients. An adult person with a communication difficulty comes to clinic with years of speaking experience, which will have brought success, failure, embarrassment, joy, comfort, rebuff and a myriad of other reactions. It is against this background that we must look at the portion of behaviour they offer us.

It was stated at the beginning of this book that intervention by a speech therapist was only justified if the person was in need and the intervention reasonably calculated to help him. It was later stated that this professional intervention could not be justified unless the person could gain help that he could not gain elsewhere. The speech therapist must be able to offer care relevant to the need. It is important to remember this as we move into areas of communicative maintenance where so many factors are involved. Examples may be helpful here. We can look at the case of Peter, cited in Chapter 1, case history 1; and of Mrs A. case history 2. It was stated in the discussion that there was possible re-interpretation on psychological/emotional grounds and we can now look at each case in this way.

Peter: The boy has two older sisters and his development has not been as swift as theirs. He therefore has a longer than usual period of verbal dependency upon females to communicate for him. He is clumsy and awkward in his movements and poorly co-ordinated. Stammering or non-fluency is evident by junior school age. At this point not only is it important that he receive linguistic help but that the consequences of his stammering behaviour are noted.

Stammer: Over protection by mother, sisters and teacher (female)

Perpetuation of stammer as an end-gaining and protective device

Ambivalence towards female dominance

Low self-esteem and ambivalent attitude towards females

Stammer: Indicative of ambivalence

or

Suppression of stammer leads to:
  Emergence of aggression and over compensatory attitudes
  Continuing difficulty in relationships with girls/women.

There are further possibilities from now on which will either improve Peter's confidence and self-esteem or further reduce it. One determinant is his own basic personality; another is his family – the attitudes of his father, mother and sisters; another is the kind of experience which he meets.

Peter could appear at a speech clinic not as a child but as an adult with any of the following complaints:

Stammer: Overt stammering with generalised communication anxiety

Stammer and personality maladjustment: Disguised Stammer with occasional interruptions of fluency only but with unhappiness and failure chronically associated with lack of ease in speaking

Clutter: Unregulated utterance but with sufficient personality strength to have coped with this. Now needs to change way of speaking because of social/job demands

Stammer: Obvious stammer but sufficient personality strength not to have been held back from accomplishment. Now wishes to change for social/domestic reasons.

The help that the speech therapist can give and the way in which she gives it will be very much determined by the complaint and the history with which she is presented.

Similarly in the case of Mrs A. there are other possibilities than that of simple voice misuse. A possible early history, taken in more detail could be this:

Childhood: Mrs A. is the only child of very elderly parents. Her father is a retired clergyman. Both he and his wife were affectionate but preoccupied with church matters during their daughter's childhood and adolescence. They were ambitious for her in that they wished her to go to university and then to take a teacher training. Her father in particular was disappointed by her refusal to do this. Mrs A. had wanted to train for a career in singing or the theatre but felt unable to carry this through in face of her parents' distress at the idea. She took a secretarial training and held good jobs subsequently but ones which gave her little outlet for creativity.

Marriage: Mr A. was one of her father's parishioners, a young accountant who has subsequently obtained a good post in Inland Revenue. The marriage has been happy. Nevertheless, Mrs A. has had periods of restlessness and depression because her life seems to be filled with 'busy work'. She regrets her early decision to train as a secretary and believes that she should either have carried through her own wishes or followed those of her parents. She has friends who have managed to pursue satisfying careers either with or without marriage and regrets that she has not explored her own talents more fully.

Mrs A. could therefore present at the speech clinic with:

Vocal dysfunction (as indicated in Chapter 1)
She is basically well adjusted but needs help in sorting out her feelings and technical help as to how to use her voice.

Hysterical aphonia
Sudden voice loss for which very slight vocal cord inflammation cannot account. This could be a hysterical condition associated with severe anxiety about some aspect of her life. She could feel unable to meet the demands placed upon her by her husband and family or by the theatrical performance in which she is engaged. There could be guilt and conflict about the time spent away from home because of her acting. Such feelings could relate back to early guilt about her feeling for acting and her parents' disapproval; they would easily be called to mind within the familiar context of church.

Mrs A's history of failing to carry through her own wishes but of taking an easier path could be seen as supporting the hypothesis of hysterical aphonia.

Spastic dysphonia
Impaired vocal quality with periods of loss. The vocal note is abnormal to an extent for which vocal cord inflammation cannot account. There is very severe and constricting tension throughout the vocal musculature. This is generally believed to be a functional disorder of a psycho-neurotic nature but has been occasionally associated with neurological impairment. If psycho-neurotic, the emotion repressed is frequently that of anger, the patient being unable to express anger and agression in an overt way. This hypothesis can be supported by Mrs A's early inability to oppose her parents. The emotion not expressed then could have been intensified by marital and domestic frustration and re-evoked by the familiar church atmosphere (for a full account of hysterical and spastic a/dysphonia see Greene, 1972). In Mrs A's case the speech therapist would appear to have less contradictory possibilities to consider than in Peter's, but in fact there are different treatment alternatives to be pursued. If the therapist attempts to promote voice use with no attention to the underlying emotions she will do her patient no service. There will be at the very least, relapse and possibly other symptoms. In both cases there is one major decision to be taken first.

'Is the speech therapist the best person to help this patient?' If it is believed that the speech or the voice is a real problem and an area of vulnerability which needs strengthening, the answer is 'yes'. If it is considered that the personality maladjustment is severe and that the voice or speech behaviour has been thrown up amongst the psycho-neurotic symptomatology, then the answer may be 'no'. But in some cases an experienced speech therapist will consider that she has something to offer even the strongly neurotic patient and will persevere in his or her aid. Most speech therapists are well advised not to attempt to change the behaviour of patients with marked psychotic tendencies.

GENERAL CONSIDERATIONS

Before looking further at particular cases we should consider failures of maintenance in the following way:
1. General difficulty in regulating and monitoring
2. Focal and precipitating circumstances

The two groups of disorders which arise out of these failures are disorders of rhythm and disorders of voicing.

In disorders of rhythm the overall regulation is the chief difficulty and therefore the main therapeutic concern. The focus which precipitates breakdown cannot always be avoided and so the person has to be strengthened in his control so that he may be better able to withstand and to recover from its ill effects. In disorders of voicing the patient is more likely to have a physical focus of laryngeal discomfort or abnormality which will need attention as well as the whole regulatory matrix. The two categories will therefore be considered separately after some discussion of regulatory processes.

Speech regulation

The conveying of ideas through the combining of speech sounds is only possible because of the organisation of activities by the brain which stems from the organisation of the brain itself. As more information percolates through from brain research, speech therapists will be forced to consider how their treatment methods can best emphasise those features which have some controlling effect on the mechanisms themselves. We have shifted from the simple concept of input and output or sensory and motor channels to appreciating that 'no line can be drawn between a sensory side and a motor side in the organisation of the brain itself' (Nauta and Feirtag, 1979). This must mean that no person with communication impairment can be assisted by an approach devoted exclusively to input or output. The gap between research into brain organisation and the effect of that research upon practitioners dealing with the effect of impairment is a very large one. Nevertheless all the major texts on speech pathology emanating from Britain or the United States in the last 15 years have found it necessary to present some model of speech function which shows how information is fed back into the mechanism during the process of utterance. The concept of feedback is now basic to speech therapy.

The early effect of the concept was simply to accentuate sensory training in cases hitherto classified as motor problems. Then we saw the creation of categories, e.g. verbal dyspraxia, which were the outcome of thinking about feedback and its disruption. Now we see a major development in the rapid growth of instrumentation which is designed to give the patient information about his performance while he is yet speaking. This is a very considerable change from the recapitulatory methods on which we have been hitherto forced to rely.

An interesting example can be seen in the method of teaching relaxation. Excessive tension of the musculature associated with anxiety has long been seen as an enemy to easy speech. It has consequently been associated with stammering and vocal dysfunction as a highly contributory if not causal activity. So relaxation to reduce excessive muscle tension and induce ease has long been part of the treatment of stammering. This treatment has been put across by contrasting the muscle sensations of tension and relaxation and encouraging the patient to feel the difference. He is then required to seek a state of relaxation by freeing himself from excessive muscle tension. This may start while he is passive, lying or sitting and then be developed to carry over into active states. Early methods of relaxation were founded on the teachings of Jacobson (1938). Many practitioners subsequently used his methods to build up their patients' tolerance of stress or at any rate their ability to respond to it in a less reactive and self punitive manner. Relaxation, however it is taught tends to constitute a philosophy as much as a technique. The methods of Alexander. (see Barlow, 1973) have introduced to many the experience of homeostasis and the resting state. Thus the patient develops the ability to maintain a balanced posture free from excessive and deforming strain while carrying out his normal activities. He is led to this state by constant experience of a correct balance which he has learnt to contrast with the imbalance and ill-health previously experienced.

The two authorities referred to and other authors besides, had to develop their methods from the contrast stimulation or the recognition of two contrasted feelings; one excessively tense and associated with anxiety; the other relaxed, well balanced and associated with ease and control. To go from one to another demanded a complete halt and then the deliberate relaxation and positioning of the body. As the disciples become more practised they are able to make the transition more swiftly and are less likely to let tension build up to intolerable limits. There are still only the two approaches to control, the first by preparing the mechanism and the second by reminding it after tension has taken place or misuse is under way.

A recent method in use with stammerers involves a relaxometer or similar apparatus which relies upon bio-feedback. The patient is given information about the state of his musculature while it is starting to contract. He does not have to wait until the adverse effects of the excessive contraction become evident in his impaired function (see Rustin, 1978). The immediacy of such devices is likely to be helpful to those who found it very difficult to develop a different state by progressive relaxation or postural re-education though it does not negate the value of these methods. Indeed a combination of the immediate and longterm may now be seen as very effective therapy for controlling excessive muscular tension.

The most successful therapy has always been that which gives the patient increasing control over his own mechanism. As research into regulatory mechanisms develops we will hope to be able to increase the control that all kinds of patients can establish over their errant mechanisms. We may also hope to see why our well proven and successful techniques have effected the improvement which occurred. We have seen much helpful work in cerebral palsy and in stammering, to name only two fields, where techniques of facilitation and regulation have been attacked because of their underlying theoretical premises but which have yet resulted in measurable progress, improvement or relief. The history of speech therapy, like that of all aspects of medicine, shows techniques and methods resurfacing in a flush of justification when the alteration of some aspect has been suggested as the result of investigation. Thus the method becomes securely based instead of being accepted as empirical medicine.

At the present time of writing there are several ideas developed in relation to computer programmes which can helpfully be used to look at speech regulation. One of these overload. If a computer is given a sudden excess of information it may break down and respond with nonsense. The mechanism it has developed for coding and stratifying or generally making use of information simply will not operate. We see such manifestations in our brain damaged patients who respond by catastrophic reaction or psychotic-type withdrawal when exposed to a sudden excess of stimulation or when given too many impressions at once. Early work, such as that of Strauss and Kephart insisted that brain damaged children must be treated in environments free from more than minimal visual stimulation in order that they could cope with organising the information they were given.

We may also see the effect of overload, not only in complete breakdown (as with an electricity circuit) but in the 'nonsense' or abnormal behaviour that starts to appear.

Some stammering can be seen in this light and evidence of it has already been suggested in these pages. The author produced a very obvious stammer in the boy Luke (see Chapter 9) during her first assessment. He was repeating after me, sentences of increasing length and complexity. Such repetition usually sheds considerable light on a person's linguistic competence in that the material will be reduced according to rules or not, once too much strain is placed upon the memory. My object being to test out Luke's memory for and recreation of language structure, I gave him sentences which were built up systematically. I then inadvertently commented upon the picture we were describing thinking that the boy would understand that my words were simply comment and not part of the task. So I said 'It's rather a nice picture don't you think?' The construction of this sentence is very different from those preceding it and the intonation much more suited to my age and disposition than his. In attempting to repeat my statement, as he believed himself required to do, Luke started with a prolonged repetition of the vowel, omitted three words, went back to retrieve them, prolonged the vowel again, repeated with tension the initial sound of the word 'nice' and allowed the final two words to trail away. Such juxtaposition of prolongation, repetition, hesitation and lack of definition in essaying an utterance is very much what is encountered in the syndrome of stammering. In this case it was the direct result of overload upon an inadequate but responsive organism.

When the speech of a normally equipped adult is exposed to stress it will show certain characteristics. Non-fluency is one of them. This may take the form of hesitation but does not usually go on to involve repetition with increasing tension nor prolongation of vowels. Slips of the tongue occur because of failure of attention or failure to process and reproduce information at speed (Boomer and Laver, 1968). There is also word finding difficulty and generally impaired efficiency in expressing thoughts in coherent, articulate speech, but this is a remediable state and does not set up a series of phenomena which become part of the speech act. There is evidence to show that language monitoring in old age is less efficient and word retrieval less speedy and accurate. This behaviour does not lead to the personality disturbances such as those associated with the phenomenon of stammering, but when stress is increased the person may show catastrophic inability to convey his thoughts to others.

We await a comprehensive neurophysiological description of linguistic processing to show us exactly how the mechanism is affected by fatigue, excitement, hormonal change or just general wear and tear. We can observe that some people are consistently fluent and well organised in their utterance and others show variation to the extent that they are not always coherent.

The variations shown by people in maintaining a functional state of language can be considered in relation to:

The strength of the mechanism itself
The kind of load it has to carry
The circumstances in which the load is carried

The brain mechanisms that handle language allow for gradual development and increase of complexity in the amount of material that can be processed. An infant is not equipped to handle more than a small number of language signals and can only respond to these signals in a limited way. As the whole mechanism develops and is perfected by use, the child can cope with a large amount of information and respond appropriately. We can therefore respond to signals coming through at speed and be able to throw out those that don't concern the message. Thus an eleven-year-old can perfectly well deal with the following; telephone rings – child answers by giving number.

Caller: 'Peter could you please find out if your mother has seen my car keys because I don't seem to have them with me'

Response: 'It isn't Peter, it's Tom and I don't think Mum's in because I heard her go out. But Dad's in the garden I think because the mower's going so if you wait I'll ask him. Have you looked in your handbag? That's where Mum always finds hers'

If we increase the input to the boy he may cope in a different way. Caller delivers the same message. Simultaneously the door bell rings and the boy's father calls him to answer the phone.

Response: 'Just hang on a minute Auntie B the door bell's gone.' (Puts down receiver and calls out:) 'it's o.k. Dad I'm answering it'. (Opens front door and sees neighbour.) 'Come in because I'm on the phone' (picks up receiver) 'right Auntie B. what do you want?'

The boys deals competently with this situation within his own scheme of priorities. As the demands increase he will be less able to cope. If the line is bad, the door bell too peremptory, his father insistent but inaudible and his friends scuffling about near the telephone we could not expect such an efficient performance. Whether each adult would approve the boy's priorities is not relevant to the argument. He has a system which allows him to cope. Had the telephone been answered by a younger child for example a different situation would have arisen.

Telephone rings – child responds by giving number slowly and clearly as she has been taught.

Caller: 'Hallo darling would you call Mummy'?
Child: 'Mummy's out'

Caller: 'Is Daddy there'?
Child: 'No'

The caller must then work through until she finds a member of the family who can cope or at least give an adequate answer. The young child is nevertheless still behaving very competently within her limits. She has interpreted the message and given an appropriate response. In summary, an organised brain can cope with a variety of messages. If too many are put in at once the brain's ability to deal with them efficiently will be impaired. Overload comes when the mechanism has to cope with a task which it is not programmed to deal with, or it may happen when the mechanism is being asked to cope with more than it can manage at one time. The messages may be coming in at an excessive rate, or the messages may be coming in at a normal rate and in a normal manner but the threshold of brain activity or programming has been affected by stress or anxiety. Consequently it cannot handle the processing or deal with its load in its usual way. If the brain mechanism for programming is already poor it cannot stand much stress. It is therefore likely to break down under a barrage of stimuli which another brain could handle without difficulty.

In discussing overload in relation to Peter and Luke, we are looking at mechanisms which have not been able to build up their language programmes systematically. We had not found a way of giving them the carefully selected input which might have allowed smooth and healthy action. Both boys were required to handle more signals than they could adequately manage. This created stress which further lowers the threshold at which breakdown was likely. The boy Luke was shown as developing some ability to handle signals at a higher level and thus use his cognitive abilities to assist him in processing information. He was developing a coding system which depended on slightly different signals or on fewer signals. While this was not adequate to all situations it did allow for function and growth. When such a system has been developed early in life and used continuously the therapist must be cautious as to the manner in which she interferes with it. Should she demand a sudden increase in the number of signals to which response must be made, she is inviting catastrophic response.

There are many adults who have built up a language system but whose neural mechanisms have not allowed them to cope with all the signals that are given them. They early develop the strategy, used eventually by Luke, of listening for content and using that for coding. They are likely to confuse words and sounds and so make speech errors or slips of the tongue which normal people only do when fatigued or under excessive stress. There are also adult speakers who do not appear able to regulate the information that they are offering. They will speak over-hurriedly and a-rhythmically so that the listener cannot understand them without repetition or additional help. Both the over-hasty speaker and the one without adequate coding mechanisms for sound can be found in the literature sometimes considered together and sometimes apart. If a person is not able to process signals in a smooth and consistent manner it is not unreasonable to expect him to have difficulty in regulating those that he himself is giving out.

Speech therapy clinics have always received a number of adults who are unable to regulate their utterance sufficiently to maintain clarity and coherence. A particular problem is seen to be in regulating speed. This population has been variously described under cluttering (Weiss, 1964), tachyphemia (Arnold, 1960) and central language imbalance (Luchsinger and Arnold, 1965). They represent the extreme of the fast uncontrolled speaking section of the normal population and whether they tip over into the abnormal depends upon the extent to which they can effect regulatory control. In some cases their difficulties as children are sufficiently conspicuous to attract the attention of medical and educational authorities. Other cases may be encountered where the child does not merit, or at any rate receive, early help and manages to cope with educational and social demands. He emerges into adult life without real awareness that he has a disorder of fluency though he realises that people do not always understand him. While occasionally irritated by being asked to speak more slowly or more clearly, he is not really disturbed by a sense of communicative or personal inadequacy. Such a case was described by the author early in her career (Fitch, 1963). In the introduction to the case it was stated that such a person 'usually comes to the speech clinic, not as the result of a recently acquired disorder, nor of any discomfort or distress of his own about his speech performance, but because other people find him difficult to understand and think it necessary that he should improve. The nature of the speech disturbance, over-hasty and inaccurate utterance, is such that the layman considers it could easily be corrected if the patient would take more care or make more effort. It is not realised that the patient is incapable of these measures because he is essentially unsure of his own speech performance and the effect of this upon others.' The description proceeds:

'*The patient*, 18 years of age, was referred to the speech therapist from the E.N.T. department. The terms of referral stated that there was no physical abnormality but that the patient spoke fast and inaccurately and people could not understand him. A subsequent report from the neurological department stated that there were no abnormal signs in the nervous system. It was considered by both the neurologist and the otolaryngologist that the patient was of above average intelligence and should benefit from speech therapy. This patient then became solely the concern of the speech therapist and the importance of the speech assessment was accordingly emphasised. Recordings of the patient's speech when played to other therapists produced widely different opinions all of which proved to be off the mark. They considered it to be:

1. Dysarthria: This was discounted because of the absence of abnormal signs in the nervous system
2. Dyspraxia: This seemed possible but not sufficiently comprehensive
3. Dyslalia associated with poor mentality: This was disproved by the patient's intellectual attainements and pursuits
4. Poor grade speech: This was discounted because it was difficult to see why a patient coming from an environment of superior speakers should not approximate to his speech environment if he had the ability.

In this patient's environment the quality of his speech must be considered defective. It was then realised that attempts to name the condition were not helpful in that they were based on insufficient examination and did not give rise to a treatment principle. The therapist considered that the descriptive term of cluttering was the most helpful designation'. We see here the difficulties of terminology to which extensive reference has already been made (Chapter 6).

The description of the case shows the youth's early strengths and weaknesses. 'The development of speech was late. Mother was uncertain as to the actual time of starting but said that he could read before he was able to speak sentences. She attributed the late speech and early reading to his time in a day nursery. The patient read fluently when he started school at 5 years. Later he went to a grammar school and did particularly well in mathematics but dropped Latin and French early. He had pronounced difficulty with spelling and was given special tuition.' 'It was intended that he should go to university, but at 16 years he was offered a job as an estimator at a paint factory. This promised to be interesting and had good prospects and the patient was adamant in choosing to accept it. The firm in question considered him to be brilliant at mathematics and generally able, but became concerned about his speech as it produced an adverse effect on others and occasionally prevented them from understanding him. It was in response to suggestions from the firm that the patient eventually came for treatment.' 'The patient at school was very good at rugby and even better at chess. He is now a county standard chess player.' Comment upon his speech from his parents showed that any difficulty in understanding him was attributed to his talking too fast. The speech analysis shows 'The first and general impression was that the speech was too fast, uncoordinated, variable and monotonous. There was a pronounced labial rhotacism and equally pronounced sigmatism varying from palatal to lateral. The lack of clarity was otherwise not related to the defective production of specific phonemes but to the extreme variability of the phonemic structure. e.g. 'fly' was pronounced with a labial plosive initially [plaɪ] and with a labial fricative initially [ɸaɪ] in the same sentence. [p] was pronounced as a bi-labial plosive initially and medially in 'puppy' and finally in 'hope' but as a bi-labial fricative in 'proper'. The assimilation was not consistent because [p] was given correct labial plosion in 'premonition' pronounced [primənɪtn] 'premonition'. 'Th' [θ] was pronounced [f] in 'thunder' and 'thousand', [d] in 'this'. 's' in addition to the usual palatal substitution was replaced by [θ] in 'seeking the secret of success', elided after the [k] in 'ecstasy', replaced by [f] in 'anxious'. [g] was articulated correctly in the word 'gome' which was the patient's pronunciation of 'gnome'. It was replaced by [b] in 'agreeable' and 'disgruntled' and by [d] in 'green'. [k was correct in 'care' and in 'curiosity'. It was replaced by a lateral fricative in 'club' but was correctly pronounced in 'Clementine'. It was replaced by a labial fricative in 'accrue' and by [ks] in 'acquisition'.

The young man had no hearing loss but severe discrimination difficulty and could only distinguish between sounds in the sibilant and fricative groups when he had been taught the sounds, in isolation for some time. Even then he was not able to identify them in words nor in nonsense words. He was unable to discriminate between [r] [l] and [j] in isolation. Nevertheless he had no difficulty in understanding speech and conversed intelligently and with spirit on a variety of subjects. Further description of the patient suggests that he had severe problems in auditory sequencing though this terminology was not employed at the time. There was also impaired diadocochinetic rate of tongue movement. He was unable to imitate any simple sound pattern of rhythm whether it was presented in melody or by tapping.

It is interesting to note that with such difficulties in recognising linguistic structure the young man had not been held back intellectually. He appeared to have learned to listen for content and meaning and was thus able to convey and receive ideas. This is characteristic of the intelligent person with auditory processing impairment. He obviously had considerable strengths and had jettisoned some of his weaknesses, e.g. foreign language learning, early in his career. He has made a good adjustment and would have been content to continue to make his own way. However, he was willing to comply with his firm's demands that he seek help though he was not enthusiastic, as he really did not know what all the fuss was about.

This puts the therapist in an interesting position. Must she create anxiety in her patient in order to alleviate it in others? Is the person himself so secure that she can afford to support him against the wishes of society or, in this case his employers? Will the mechanism stand up to stress or is there any indication that overload could lead to breakdown?

'During any period of listening and sound imitation the patient appeared distressed and strained. He would screw up his eyes or stare into space. Ability to imitate a simple intonation pattern was poor and together with singing produced very effortful and painful grimaces and eye screwing. During assessment and subsequent treatment the patient was co-operative but showed a lack of ease and certainty. At any point of failure or breakdown in his ability to produce or reproduce sounds he showed a mild catastrophic reaction.'

It appears more than possible then that this mechanism will not stand up to stress and the patient's only hope without therapy is to avoid putting himself into stressful situations. This cannot and should not be suggested to a young man of 18 and so, given the same choice some twenty years later I would certainly advocate treatment. My recommendations then were that treatment should be:

1. To arouse interest in the sounds of speech
2. To improve auditory attention and memory for sound and for tune and rhythm
3. To encourage the patient to rely more on auditory information and less on visual
4. To encourage him to understand and appreciate the effect of speech upon other people
5. To maintain his co-operation throughout the entire procedure by giving him specific tasks wherever possible
6. To draw his attention to the sounds which are most consistently deviate and mispronounced ('r' and 's') and to bring these nearer

to their accepted phoneme, thereby to reduce the amount of assimilation in contiguous sounds.

In deciding at this point how such a person might be helped we may set out:

Therapeutic procedures:

To affirm that a problem exists

To demonstrate the nature of the problem to the patient

To analyse the speech performance with the patient

To arouse his interest in the nature of speech sounds and of contrasting features

To improve auditory sequential skills

To maintain his co-operation and interest by working within a suitable frame of reference.

To expand the last therapeutic aim; it is no use trying to coerce an unwilling adult to adapt himself to other people's requirements if he believes the requirements to be unreasonable. To say to this young man 'You must pronounce the 's' sound correctly because it will make a better impression on prospective employers' places the therapist immediately in the category of the unreasonable or the excessively middle class. To present him with factual information upon the incidence of the sound 's' in the English language and then to show the occasions when it could critically affect meaning is a much better selling point. Anyone with a mathematical, logical mind could well be attracted to the systematic representation of sounds in their language. If, of course, the young man was able to work out that his chances of being understood were mathematically greater than the chances of being misunderstood the therapist would have to concede victory. The point to be made however is that speech change should not be a matter of moral exhortation but one subject to intelligent appraisal on both sides.

The position would be very different if the young man had himself sought treatment at a later stage when he had already broken down under stress. Although he seems able to withstand some of the demands of his environment he is suggested as being at risk and, granted an increase of pressure might not be able to withstand it.

The clutterer already described should now be considered as having already been given a responsible job which depended on communicative ability. He has the same reported problem with certain sounds and the same reported difficulty in perceiving what he is doing and how it differs from conventional speech. In the attempt to make himself clear he is forced into more and more circumlocutions. This is fatiguing and its effects are accumulative. He starts to avoid speaking situations and relies on other people to carry out some of his responsibilities. He therefore becomes more anxious because he is not pulling his weight. We thus have the start of a circle of anxiety which may break down fluency. If he comes to the speech clinic he will have increased motivation to improve but will also have anxiety which may exacerbate his symptoms even with the therapist and prevent calm analysis. So the procedure must start differently.

Therapeutic focus:

Relieve anxiety by defining the problem

Choose one element of the speech which can be changed fairly easily, e.g. show placement for 'f' and 'θ' and teach the latter

Discuss immediate strategies for self-help and presentation.

Here the therapist must try to help the whole mechanism to become more efficient by reducing the anxiety which creates the stress under which it is labouring. If she cannot do that the patient will not be able to learn. The juxtaposition of methods of reducing stress and methods of improving competence is part of all therapeutic procedure for patients with regulatory or maintenance problems. They thus constitute a large element in the literature of disorders of fluency and maintenance.

In the case just cited there was marked difficulty in monitoring through the auditory channel and such is the characteristic picture in cluttering. Auditory information is received after the speech event and thus the person cannot change his position for articulation or reject a word previously selected without stopping the flow of speech. If he is not receiving adequate auditory feedback he will have no reason to stop and re-position the articulators or offer a new word in place of one used in error. The emphasis on slowing down the speed of the clutterer, which is almost invariably placed, is so that he may have time to make such accommodations. If he has not achieved control over patterning, rhythm, sequencing and pausing he will not be able to start to do so unless his speech can be slowed down. Once the speed is reduced by phrasing or syllable timing, the underlying language structures can be investigated in more detail. It will then be found how much the excessive rate has caused the impaired linguistic imbalance.

Considerations in the literature vary from those which place great emphasis upon speed regulation and those which incline towards linguistic restructuring. Both methods must however rely upon the clutterer being able to obtain more information about his performance.

If it is decided to go for basic rate and rhythm before changing articulatory placement the therapist may proceed in the following way:

Training foci:

Relaxation: reducing the degree of muscle tension thus slowing down reaction rate and creating sensations of ease.

Imitation: of vocal cadence with simple intonation; of intonation patterns with more complicated timing. Both can involve the laryngograph.

Auditory training: This is part of the above procedure and can be carried on without the visual trace once some proficiency has been attained. The clutterer can practice on his own using a loop recording with the therapist's model utterance pre-recorded. From this point the cluttering patient must start to initiate and record his own phrases using the same stress patterns as those he has been practising but providing his own words. Thus:

Therapist's model:

First utterance: I'm going out

Second utterance: I'm coming back again

Third utterance: I'm going out but I'm coming back again.

Clutterer's utterance

First: He's coming back

Second: He's going out again

Third: He's coming back but he's going out again.

Dialogue

Therapist: I'm going out but I'm coming back again

Clutterer: He's coming back but he's going out again.

The dialogue would be practised first with a pause between the speakers and then the clutterer would be required to cut in sooner but still control his rate once started.

The nearer the therapist can work to colloquial speech the more likely she is to assist her patient maintain control. It is tempting to use poetry reading and recitation to develop a sense of rhythm, but this gives little feedback to the patient on how to monitor his own utterance. He is more likely to make this connection if natural speech is used.

If production difficulties have not been ironed out by working on rate and rhythm they must now be attacked, but here other monitoring channels must be used in addition to auditory. Tactile and proprioceptive feedback are both used to monitor placement. Tactile feedback is normally received as the position is adopted. Proprioceptive feedback operates just before the utterance. It may therefore be more helpful to the clutterer to separate these channels and work on placement, precision and speed of movement without using sound. Then sound may be reintroduced in the form of underlying vocalization, and then of varied patterns with voiced, whispered and stressed speech all represented.

Dalton and Hardcastle in their valuable discussion of disorders of fluency (1977) examine the effect of co-articulation upon the clutterer's phonology and point out that the co-articulation is induced both by speed and by lack of constraint at word and syllable boundaries. These points suggest that both reduced speed and awareness of linguistic structure must be promoted. Auditory training may therefore be graded so that the clutterer not only listens for sounds in different positions in words (as in the well established discrimination procedures) but has to listen to them in segments which show right left or left right influence. He should then practise aloud words and phrases – e.g. indoors; in there – and use them in his practice of longer utterances. Once he recognises the changes that are important in speech he should be encouraged to record narrative of increasing length and excitement and then go back with his check list to see when control started to slip. As Hardcastle and Dalton point out, it should soon be possible to alert the clutterer to his increasing rate by some bio-feedback device so that he is not totally dependent upon retrospective action. Such devices have, as has been stated, been successfully employed with stammerers.

Stammering or stuttering

This has been the subject of so much research and experiment that there is little need to give a further account here of its symptomatology. Relevant texts will be cited in the bibliography.

The term stammering refers to many forms of behaviour and these are now thought to stem for a number of causes. Most stammerers show distress and anxiety associated with the act of speech as the result of long experience of failure and embarrassment. It is generally believed that these attitudes in themselves predispose the stammerer to further interruptions of his fluency and thus perpetuate it. Treatment methods therefore involve both exploration of attitudes and symptom control. Literature on the subject suggests that a large number of approaches have been found useful.

Discussion has failed to determine however whether methods have succeeded because they are intrinsically valuable in themselves or because they introduce a positive element into a speech situation which is suffused with anxiety and negativism. At this point we can still say that every method helps some people and no one method helps everyone. Good therapy in stammering, as in cerebral palsy and aphasia depends outstandingly on a well ordered approach related to a pervasive but practical philosophy. In cases cited in these pages the child has been shown to be vulnerable is some way during language acquisition and so may break down if too much is demanded of him. In some cases he will break down into language disorder but in others, such as that of the child Benjamin (Chapter 8) he is at risk of continuing to stammer and with increased severity. The growth of stammering from initial non-fluency is strongly represented in the literature notably by Wendell Johnson and Van Riper.

If stammerers present themselves at the speech clinic as adults they are likely to have years of stammering behind them. Onset in adult life is so a-typical as to merit full psychiatric and neurological investigation. The speech therapist must have something to offer any person she takes on for treatment and when she is dealing with a longstanding complaint of such a complex nature she must be particularly realistic and honest in what she offers.

It was suggested in Chapter 2 that there were basic skills that the speech therapist must have in order to effect a change for the better in her patients. It was stated that the condition of stammering might need the *modification of behaviour*: This will be based upon careful observation of the act of stammering. The act may include eye blinking, sweating, laryngeal constriction, altered breathing rate, concomitant movements, averted gaze, prolongation, circumlocution, repetition, spasm of articulatory or laryngeal musculature. It may simply be manifested in repetition and hesitation on comparatively few words. If therapy based upon behaviour modification with reward, punishment, cancellation and reinforcement is used, decisions must first be made as to the target behaviour which is to be changed. The choice of this method will also demand intensive therapy since behaviour cannot be altered except on a highly systematic basis. Therapists using this method are advised to have particular training themselves since it is a powerful tool and one that must be thoroughly understood.

Attention training: This is likely to be a necessary adjunct to many methods as stammerers have had their communicative energy siphoned off into their own performance. They have frequently stopped paying attention and listening to other people because of the excessive speech anxiety and self absorbtion consequent upon it.

Listening: In addition to being encouraged to listen to the speech of other people stammerers have also been given techniques of re-training which are based on listening rather than speaking. These include modelling and shadowing where the stammerer listens and repeats what is said at a prescribed rate and manner. This can be associated with relaxation.

Control over movement patterns: The stammerer performs many movements during the act of speech which are not part of the normal act and which can therefore distract him and others and generally add to the overwhelming discomfort felt by both speaker and listener. The movements that are not necessary for smooth utterance should be the target of specific relaxation and control.

Imitation: This is used continually by the therapist to allow the stammerer to experience a sense of fluency. As stammering occurs more often and more severely in self-initiated speech the therapist may hope to use imitation to gain control over some elements. It relieves the stammerer of having to think of his own words and allows him to concentrate on the smooth performance of a simple utterance. It is also used to encourage deliberate stammering or repetition, in syllable timed utterance, with the metronome and in a very large number of other ways by which the therapist offers a model.

Relaxation: This has been used in the treatment of stammerers in this country since the early days of the profession of speech therapy. In the school speech clinics of the forties and fifties small boys could be found lying on mats specially provided for the purpose while therapists described soothing scenes to them. There was then usually a period of complete silence while the child (or adult) was encouraged to direct his attention to different parts of his body to reduce tension and thence to attain an overall state of calm. This was frequently followed by easy speech with rhythmic utterances and often strong suggestion ('every day in every way, I am getting better and better'). Differential relaxation on the lines of Jacobson and overall retraining on the Alexander principle have already been referred to in this chapter. However relaxation is taught it must surely play some part in the management of people with a high degree of anxiety. It has already been pointed out that anxiety, by creating stress and hypertonicity in the musculature, will affect the way in which the speech mechanism can deal with signals and generate signals itself. So to reduce the rate at which signals create reactions is in the interest of all disfluent patients and this can be done by systematic relaxation. But, anxiety cannot be maintained at a reduced level unless the person can learn to behave more effectively in the feared situation. We therefore see:

Relaxation plus suggestion

Relaxation with de-sensitisation
Relaxation and easy speech or deliberate stammering
Relaxation and anticipation or pre-planning
Relaxation followed by rehearsal.

We then see a swing by which the feared situation is tackled head on as it were. The stammerer is encouraged to discuss his fears so that the situation is robbed of something of its terror. This is essentially abreactive in effect and may be followed *by relaxation associated with insight.*

Such methods were the speech therapists stock in trade for many years. At the present time we are drawn to symptom control in the first instance to give the adult patient some relief. This gains his confidence in the therapist and restores his confidence in himself. When a technique of fluency has been achieved in propitious surroundings the work is on to maintain its use. At this point attitudes and fears may be discussed and conditioning procedures adopted. The therapist whether she starts with feelings and goes on to function, or starts with function and goes on to feelings, is responsible for the whole spectrum and can no more abandon her patient when she has taught him to relax than she can give him a technique of fluency and leave him to inspire his own confidence in its use.

Recently much interest has been shown in Britain in a masking device which prevents the stammerer hearing his own voice (Dewar and Dewar, 1976). This device was developed in accordance with experimental evidence which showed that stammering was influenced by the stammerer's auditory feedback. The masking device has certainly yielded considerable relief to many and it is for therapists trained in its use to add the necessary support and practice which will enable those using it to achieve long term benefit. Any device which offered instant fluency used to be eyed askance by speech therapists whose clinics were quickly filled with those relapsing from its effects. As our knowledge of feedback and the mechanisms by which monitoring is thus controlled become more exact, we may hope to see adjuncts to therapy which capitalise on this knowledge and become of permanent value.

A device previously used with enthusiasm in Britain was that of the electronic metronome which aimed to establish the basic timing pulse which the disfluent patient lacked. Wohl summarising her paper on the subject (1968) stated that 'fluent speech requires that a firm matrix of language and speech patterns be laid down; that a complete blue-print of speech activity be designed before utterance is commenced and that the mechanism be capable of organising the temporal distribution of stimuli. Among the influences which can inhibit the formation of the matrix are slow or irregular neuromuscular maturation, insufficient or unacceptable language stimulation, failure to equate visual and auditory feed-in, delay in feedback and misinformation or lack of feedback information.

It is suggested therefore that choice of focus depends upon this inadequacy of the matrix when neurovegetative influences, failure of the suppressor or inhibitory mechanisms, morbidity of the neuromuscular system, failure of the timing mechanisms and synaptic delay or other erratic influence are brought to bear.'

The therapist cannot escape her role of diagnostician even when the person presents himself with a disturbance of fluency or rhythm which has for centuries been called *stammering*. She must consider the matrix and the focus devising therapy to support the one and reduce the effects of the other. She must remember the history of anxiety and despair and offer hope; she must remember the history of deception and disillusionment and offer realistic counsel. She must contrive to create the propitious framework for her treatment whether it be a large group or an individual session. Familiarity has not bred contempt for this crippling handicap but we are getting much better at cutting it down to size.

Nevertheless the author remembers with some amusement being asked to take part in a television programme with the reassurance "Don't worry about it. We will just ask you something easy like 'what is stammering'?"

Disorders of rhythm and fluency have been offered under the general framework of regulation and maintenance. The choice of the last two terms indicates that for the patient and for the therapist the process of change is gradual and needs regular attention. If dramatic changes are seen and these for the better, both patient and therapist must reinforce them by persistent effort. If the change is for the worse effort must again be made to determine what went wrong and to rebuild the processes of control. The stammerer or stutterer has been previously unable to regulate and maintain smooth, rhythmic utterance. He works to achieve this by controlling the timing of his signals as well as he can and by preventing himself being overcome with the panic which will throw up old reactions. The therapist also offers endurance and persistence, matching the stammerer in these respects and giving him stalwart but not uncritical support. In this way he can develop more insight and can also relax his guard in order to learn more about himself. If the game becomes too easy for him and he is cruising along with a captive audience while he is tempted only to expand upon himself and not to change, then the therapist must take on the role of mentor instead of mother and give a few stringent reminders about the purpose of their meetings.

The same injunctions apply whenever the therapist is working with people who have a strong initial need for reassurance. It is a difficult shift for an inexperienced therapist to make and she is more likely to persist overlong in a reassuring role than to remind the patient of his responsibilities to himself and her. This is why an experienced colleague is so helpful. She may be able to see more easily how little one party or the other is actually contributing to therapy. Or if both are contributing but progress appears at a standstill she may be able to make a suggestion which will increase understanding on both sides and take the treatment a step further. Many stammerers benefit from meeting with more than one therapist, the first as group director and the second as individual instructor. Such juxtaposition prevents the two personalities becoming so comfortably adjusted that no growth can take place because there is no friction.

Voicing

Disorders of voicing can also be seen within the categories of maintenance and regulation. Normal voice production depends on smooth, synergistic action of small and large muscle groups and is maintained by auditory and proprioceptive feedback. Good voice production to fit the voice for extra demand is based upon breath capacity and control, relaxation and good posture, flexible movements of the articulators and well placed forward tone. The use of such phrases as 'forward tone' reminds us that most precepts used in vocal training depend upon imagination rather than insight. Singing teachers have exhorted their pupils to 'float the voice upon the breath' to produce 'white' notes and 'dark' notes and 'silver' notes. Gounod is said to have asked a singer to produce a 'dark purple note' and when asked for further elucidation replied 'the sort of sound you can wash your hands in'.

Two attempts have been made in Britain to develop an exact and scientific means of classifying vocal behaviour. The plan by Laver was first published in 1968 as a componential descriptive model and has since been developed by that author into a more comprehensive index (in press.) One of Laver's objects was to construct an index which could be used for reference by several professions; speech therapists, phoneticians, psychologists and psychiatrists. Wynter, publishing in 1974, tried to determine what degree of conformity was to be found in groups of speech therapists and students in assigning labels and degrees of severity to vocal states. Listeners were asked to make their judgements from recordings. This study has also been developed and it is hoped that it will offer some scale on which severity of vocal conditions can be rated. By such means we hope to approach the position, already held in language, where information and evaluation can be made and passed on to colleagues without change. Some rating scales also exist for fluency but none, as yet for vocal disorders. Assessment of vocal dysfunction remains a very individual business though it need not be entirely subjective. We now have sufficiently sensitive instruments to record volume and pitch change though these are not always available to practicing clinicians. It is important that some measures of vocal state and vocal change be made so that progress can be charted.

Whereas the stammerer may be helped most in a group of fellows the voice patient will almost certainly need careful individual therapy that starts with a meticulous voice examination. This will not be carried out until the patient has seen the laryngologist. There are many organic and neuropathological causes to voice breakdown but we are not concerned with those in this chapter. Such conditions are well described in Greene (1972) and Boone (1980), as indeed are the functional voice disorders which will be the main focus of this discussion. They are included here however because it is believed that they can be seen in relation to regulatory and maintenance procedures previously introduced.

Voice maintenance
This is not normally considered very seriously, as it is taken for granted that the normal human instrument can stand up to the normal demands placed upon it. These demands do not vary very much once a routine of living is established, but if extra demand is combined with other factors, such as infection, inflammation, fatigue, excessive tension or hormonic imbalance, then the person may find his, or in these cases usually her, voice giving trouble. The trouble is then frequently exacerbated by the behaviour of the person in any attempt to produce more volume. A smoker, suffering slight laryngeal irritation, temporarily combined with extreme general fatigue, may suddenly have to cope with the visit of a deaf, elderly relative. The burden of work is increased adding to the fatigue and the amount of vexing occurrences in the household will almost certainly rise. All this adds to the desire to smoke with a consequent increase in laryngeal irritation. The need to speak more loudly to a deaf person will be likely to produce vocal misuse by effort. This ordinary domestic overload can be seen time

and time again but of course it does not by any means qualify the sufferer for immediate voice therapy unless concern and discomfort are very great. Whether the problem disappears or goes on to become habitual will depend on how each element is tackled. The person may stop smoking and relieve the initial irritation. The household may settle down and she will get more rest. She will become used to communicating with her elderly relative or get him a hearing aid. Another member of the family will be more helpful and relieve the burden. An element of self-punishment is taken out of the sufferer's behaviour.

Looked at in another way the position could deteriorate. The sources of frustration and anger increase; the person's own health deteriorates; other small irritations are added which she could normally ride over but which now become major targets. The voice trouble is offered to the family as a sign of the burden on its chief buttress and becomes a major signal for help. It is because the balance of emotion, misuse, foolish behaviour and deep underlying feeling is so delicate in all of us that the therapist cannot give out superficial advice without very careful investigation. In the case just described there is need for straight forward and sympathetic discussion of the very natural feelings that may be contributing to fatigue and frustration. There may subsequently be need to explore attitudes and feelings at a deeper level and help the patient to show more tolerance toward herself or to develop more insight into what she is doing to herself and others. Vocal training will be devoted towards restoring useful healthy function rather than increasing the range of the instrument. Emphasis on health will include advice about sources of irritation (the E.N.T. surgeon may already have emphasised this) and then practical demonstration and practice as to how to produce notes without strain. Emphasis can then be placed on clear articulation to allow communication with a deaf person without the need to shout. In summary

Training foci:

Relaxation coupled with encouragement to express feelings

Vocal hygiene: explanation of vocal mechanism and how it functions

Voice production: emphasis on well produced note and good articulation

Ear training: to perceive the slight changes which can indicate misuse.

} Feedback

If necessary the therapist will enlist medical help to relieve real depression or improve general health.

We may now consider vocal manifestations that arise over a long period of time but with increasing frequency and in such a way as to suggest an underlying weakness. This may be located in the larynx as in the cases described by Greene under 'hyperkinetic dysphonia' and Boone under 'hyerfunction'. The tension in the vocal cords is inappropriate to the activity demanded. The patient may have been speaking for years on an unsuitable pitch which can only be maintained by excessive tension in the laryngeal and pharyngeal muscles. This tension has spread to the muscles of the shoulders and back and subsequently to the intercostals, abdominal muscles and diaphragm. The patient habitually uses an excess of energy to maintain even an ordinary vocal activity like simple conversation. As she is already at the high peak of tension no additional demand can be yielded too. Attempts to sing or to project the voice therefore lead to pitch cracks and fluctuations or to intermittent dysphonia.

It would seem to be a simple matter to persuade someone like this to reduce some of the tension associated with speaking. The course of treatment would appear to be:

Relaxation

Ear training: to discern pitch change and to note stridency

Breath control: based on relaxed and reciprocal muscle action

Local relaxation and placement of the articulators which are likely to be tense and retracted

In fact the initial step, of persuading someone to free herself of an approach to life which may have characterised her for twenty or more years is far from simple. We carry our protective tensions around with us like armour. We feel vulnerable and exposed without them and if suddenly required to drop this guard may feel at a loss as to how to function at all. The therapist may therefore choose to change her order of procedures:

Training foci:

Vocal production: contrast between initiating voice with harsh and soft attack

Ear training: associated with the above

Bio-feedback: to give additional information associated with above

OR

Vocal exercises: extended into continuous speech

Use of laryngograph to practice smooth trace.

At this point the patient may be starting to perceive that excessive tension is not efficient in voice production and may be prepared to question its efficiency elsewhere. Such procedure is comparable to the sympton control initially taught to the stammerer. An effective demonstration can improve confidence and make future suggestions as to change easier for the patient to accept. It also provides another way in which to support the patient for if symptom control is not effective the attitudes and tensions that are producing the symptom may expose themselves for discussion.

The range of functional voice disorders is from the straight misuse to the revelation of neurosis and deep seated personality disturbance (See bibliography). The therapist needs allies and professional help in training herself to deal with this range. Her own needs include *thorough knowledge of the voice: how it functions and how it can be controlled.*

We may here return to Chapter 2 of this book where there was some discussion of the therapist's voice. In the early stages of speech therapy training the student was required to spend several hours a week on her own voice. This meant training herself in

Capacity and control of breathing
Control of pitch and extension of pitch range
Improved resonance and tone
Flexibility and control of the organs of articulation.

The object of this work was to give the student thorough knowledge of how the instrument worked and how it could be maintained and used. Unfortunately (in the opinion of this author) such requirements are no longer made. The student's range of theoretical study and her need for clinical practice is now so great that there is no time for her own vocal training. It is suggested that she acquire the requisite vocal ability by some other means than regular supervised instruction by the staff of her training school or university department. It is questionable whether this can be done. There are moreover other factors to be considered. Vocal training has long been reckoned to be a middle and professional class luxury. The present re-examination of the therapist's role rejects such a background as the only basis for admission. It is to be hoped that some means of restoring vocal training, free from its earlier identification will be made in the future. If so it will give the student extremely valuable working knowledge about vocal function which she cannot acquire any other way. She will have a built in model and is therefore confident in her ability to show the patient what is required without being dependent upon mechanical apparatus.

Counselling and psychotherapy

The limits of the speech therapist's and psychiatrist's domain are ill charted in the area of aphonia and dysphonia. A not unusual progress is for the young therapist to start by dealing with cases of habitual misuse and organically based dysphonias. As she becomes more experienced she may start to retain those patients whom she previously referred to the psychiatrist. This will come about because of their own working relationship and the psychiatrist's willingness to act as resource but not to carry the whole burden of management. Such co-operation is extremely valuable in cases where the patient is abusing the voice and needs local retraining but where the underlying personality needs are too severe to be met by symptom control. There is no intention here to relegate the speech therapist to a technical assistant but rather to point out that the mechanisms of conversion hysteria, psychosis, depression or acute anxiety are the professional territory of the psychiatrist and need his care. There will be many patients where the anxiety and guilt can be contained by the voice therapist and where she remains in charge of the case. The point is well discussed in texts already referred to and in books cited in the bibliography.

Working relations with the E.N.T. department is the largest factor in the extension of the speech therapist's experience in voice work. The best results are always obtained when she has constant access to this department and can be present during laryngological examination (Bull and Cook, 1976). In some cases the relationship between the vocal and laryngeal state is extremely close; in others it is very loose indeed. Both specialists need help in puzzling out the relationship in these latter instances. Ready access to the medical department concerned will give the speech therapist information on health, hearing and specific diseases which may be entirely relevant to her treatment and which she will otherwise have to seek out at a cost of the patient's time and sometimes of his confidence. However once the condition has been thoroughly evaluated there may be everything to be said for treating the patient elsewhere. As was pointed out in Chapter 4 the association with a medical atmosphere might have a depressing effect on some patients and reinforce a suggestion overtly contradicted, that there was a medical problem which for most people would suggest cancer.

If, however, voice disorders are assessed and treated in a hospital department as a matter of routine the association with cancer may be diminished. The work of one such department has been described by Simpson (1971) and Simpson, Helman and Gordon (1975). All patients with voice disorders seen at the Dysphonic Clinic of the Department of Otolaryngology, Victoria Infirmary, Glasgow, receive comprehensive medical examination and then special investigations, involving tomography and cine-radiography.

They co-operate in stroboscopic and aerodynamic studies, the nature of which is carefully explained to them. Emphasis is therefore placed on exact and scientific knowledge of laryngeal function, clinical and phonatory. Patients examined in this manner therefore view the department more positively than if its sole purpose is to identify disease. It is greatly to be hoped that other departments of otolaryngology will extend their facilities in this way so that patients may be similarly treated and students appropriately trained.

11

Disorders following a change of state

There remain to be considered all those patients who have been robbed of their power to speak as they did formerly because of some permanent affliction or change of state. The needs of this group are very different from those we have discussed earlier. We have seen that developmental disorders in children may interfere with their emotional, social and educational progress and we wish to give assistance as early as possible so that the child may gain command over language, preferably by means of normal speech. We have also considered some of those adults who remain vulnerable or at a disadvantage in a swiftly speaking society. In these cases the speech therapist gives support and re-training to enable the most efficient and pleasant function to be maintained.

The demands made by sudden deprivation of spoken language are of a different kind. In some instances the affliction is such that the speech therapist meets her patient first in a speechless state. In other cases there has been a mild or moderate change in the manner in which the patient is able to communicate. He may not be able to convey his ideas clearly or accurately but he can get across a great deal of information and in so doing express much of himself. Even if the change is so slight as to be predominantly apparent to the speaker and not to his family or associates, he will certainly be affected in the way he deals with his life. A sudden change in a skill, hitherto taken for granted is always frightening. It brings home the realisation of mortality, the very little control any person has over his life and the extent to which his view of himself depends upon a certain efficiency in making statements, forming relationships or perhaps possessing 'a talent to amuse'. There will therefore be a basic state of disquiet in any person with speech deterioration and this may move to profound distress or despair if the deterioration is severe or if his life has been built upon the skill of speaking. In most instances the speech therapist will be ignorant of the way in which her patient spoke pre-morbidly. She will not know how much he prizes verbal communication, how much he delights in words, puns, quips and general conversation. Yet she must try to help him re-build his life so that he can still realise himself as a person. It is here that the imaginative insight, indicated as being essential to the speech therapist, will be so much required. If the therapist does not understand how her patient wishes to speak and how he used to speak she will not be able to persuade him to work towards recovery nor yet to adapt his fragmented utterance. Neither will she be able to assess the extent of the trauma sustained by him and the effect upon his family and his associates. Without something of this knowledge any rehabilitation may seem mechanical or even insensitive.

In addition to this imaginative speculation the speech therapist must have the most exact information possible as to the condition which has affected or is continuing to affect the patient. Medical co-operation is essential. The speech therapist must seek out the relevant medical consultant in order to be sure that she has this essential knowledge. Adults do not suddenly lose control of a skill enjoyed and practised for many years unless there is some pathological cause. Knowledge of this cause will ensure that the most appropriate management is carried out. Ignorance of the cause may not only interfere with this management but could lead to active mismanagement with severe effects upon the patient's well-being. There are three broad categories of pathology which may be involved.

Localised organic or neurological change

Central neurological change

Psychiatric breakdown.

These categories are not discrete and must also be considered as either non-progressive, slowly or rapidly progressive. The speech therapist must have recourse to the neurologist, otolaryngologist, psychiatrist or geriatrician to determine whether she has anything to offer.

Having emphasised the importance of medical knowledge it is next helpful to recall, by means of diagrammatic representation, what the likely effects will be upon language (Fig. 3 on page 208).

Although the same model may be used as for the child it must be considered in a different way. One outstanding difference is in the relative importance of the sensory input. *Hearing* is basic to the child's acquisition of language. Without it the brain will not receive the information which allows it to sort out the linguistic code, nor yet to acquire the rich symbolism which nourishes thought. Sudden loss of hearing in adult life will have severe emotional effects but the effect upon speech will be one of deterioration only in mainte-

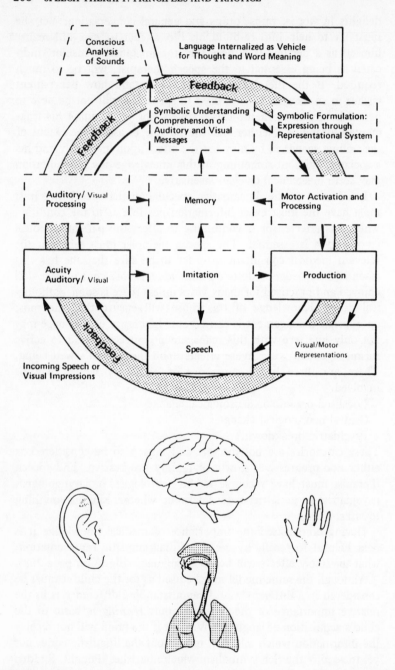

Fig. 3 (repeat)

nance. The person already possesses the reserve or language store which can generate ideas and he may express or respond to these ideas through another medium than speech. *Blindness* will cause tragic loss of independence initially but should not lead to deterioration of spoken language as this can be monitored by the normal feedback mechanisms and the person can receive plenty of communicative stimulation through listening.

Looking laterally along the diagram we can see that is easier for an adult to compensate for production difficulty than it is for a child. He will have long memory of putting messages into vocal and articulate effect and this may automatically result in his producing some elements of the message correctly. He may make minor accommodations as was suggested in Chapter 2, to clarify or to emphasise aspects of speech rendered difficult by his condition, and he will draw upon his language store to generate new ways of expressing himself if old ones fail. So acquired oro-facial or laryngeal abnormality should not render an adult speechless in a total way although it may radically affect his voice or his articulation.

As we move up the hierarchical representation the more profound and pervasive difficulties can be seen. At the *auditory* and *motor processing* level true language starts to be threatened. The patient cannot make sense of a message heard nor adequately assemble an answer. If he retains good intellectual or cognitive/symbolic functioning he may be able to receive and convey meaning by other representations, but these are likely to be limited and unsatisfactory and will leave the patient very much at risk in society. If he loses access to his word store, or his ability to retrieve words, he is even more handicapped because he cannot find other representations to compensate. In these areas there is catastrophic interference with what Professor Quirk has described as 'the almost mystical relationship between the person and the language he speaks'. This affliction is not made easier to bear because it is not easily apparent to others. Even if accompanied by other neurological signs, such as hemiplegia, which suggest that the patient has some physical cause for his affliction, he may remain a mystery to other people because of the inconsistent way he uses and responds to speech and this leads them to suspect mental rather than neurological deterioration.

If the thought processes are impaired by conditions of organic dementia the patient cannot be expected to respond to speech therapy. Psychotic incoherence or disturbance in the thought/word

process as with schizophrenia does not have the same basis in cortical degeneration and causes of these conditions are not fully
known. Such patients are not usually referred to the speech therapist. If they do come into her care it is likely to be the result of
misdiagnosis rather than intention. The speech therapist has a
rehabilitatory role with adults and must obviously apply it where
rehabilitation is at least a fair possibility. The patient who presents
himself for this treatment wishes to be as he was before. If he cannot achieve this he may accept a diminished level of function but he
will still have his own goals and these should be the goals of the
therapist also:

To be able to speak intelligibly

To be able to express himself and maintain his personality

To be able to communicate effectively

To be independent, or as independent as possible.

The extent to which any patient can succeed in achieving these
goals is not just dependent upon his basic condition nor yet upon
the skilled therapy available to him. The determining factors are
likely to be his own personality and the support he receives from
his family. In the event of gradual loss of hearing there may be
gradual adaptation even though the patient and his family do not
find it easy to come to terms with the increasing disability. If the
sufferer is reasonably robust psychologically and yet sensitive to
other people, he will be able to maintain his communicative skills
without too much professional assistance. If he is excessively sensitive and subject to mistrust and depression his state will be very
different. If the hearing loss is suddenly and traumatically
occasioned the demands on the patient's spiritual and psychological
resources and those of his family will be very suddenly made and
therefore very severely tested. There may be initial rallying with
gradual diminution of support or there may be initial shock and
confusion with subsequent insight. The prognosis for communication depends on the long term rather than the immediate attitudes
but if the immediate reaction from the family is supportive and
loving it creates a momentum of care which the speech therapist
may extend.

These same considerations will occur again when contemplating
the likely prognosis for communication in other patients. The
speech therapist is wise to try to determine how she may promote
the most constructive attitudes. She must not be beguiled into
thinking adults are not depressed because they are jovial and matter
of fact at initial interview. Nor must she assume that family relationships will not be helpful simply because they are not expressed

in the way that she personally has come to associate with love and acceptance. The way in which different members of a family view each other, the extent to which they need and value each other and the way they can support each other have been built upon years of personal adaptation and cultural and temperamental dictates. It is not easy for an outside person confronted with a sudden catastrophe, to appreciate the true feelings of everyone concerned. The therapist must do the best she can, taking the lead in explaining the handicap and the methods of rehabilitation but allowing the members of the family to absorb and react to it in their individual ways. If, as she becomes more acquainted with the family she comes across attitudes which are unhelpful or harmful she must of course try to minimise their effects if not to change them, but it is wise to start with the practicalities. If you start by showing a wife how to adapt her speech to her husband's sudden loss of hearing it will soon become apparent whether she has any real interest in doing so. At this point more intensive counselling may be given, but there are many instances where the effect of handicap is so profound that unless counselling at a deep and personal level is given early no adaptation can be made by either party.

It is not possible therefore to convey in one facile exposition the levels of feeling which are encountered by adults who have suddenly been faced with a profound change in their lives. The experienced therapist will at least know that many levels of reaction should be looked for. The inexperienced therapist should seek to build up her own counselling and supportive skills by taking additional courses and by reading as well as by attentive study of individual cases. She will find additional training in counselling extremely helpful in working with patients with acquired aphasia. Because the patient reasonably views his time with the speech therapist as his time to speak, he may discuss with her all sorts of personal difficulties or worries which he finds himself unable to get across when he sees his doctor or the consultant. The physical conditions of hospital out-patients do not usually facilitate confidential discussion. Moreover the consultant is nearly always working against the clock and dysphasic speech takes time to unravel. Even if the wife or husband is there to put the points, the patient may not wish to open up the subject. So the speech therapist may be told things that pertain to marital or sexual problems or to specific medical changes in the patient's condition. She must be able to give time and assistance where she can and to pass the information on rapidly where it is important that she should do so. If the anxiety is over the patient's medical condition she must refer to the doctor in charge of the case. If the matter is an emotional or sexual one the decision is not so clear. Several speech therapists have preferred to take additional training so that they may assist here and prevent the aphasic person having to relate to another person a matter he finds embarassing and which his dysphasia makes it extremely difficult for him to speak about. Other speech therapists believe that their relationship with the patient is best centred in speech and language and that it is easier for them both if personal and marital difficulties are discussed elsewhere. The decision should be an individual one, made by the speech therapist in the light of her experience and training. Once more the support of a senior colleague may be invaluable in reaching the decision.

The speech therapist should never be working alone but she frequently occupies a unique position, as indeed she should. A handicapped adult will need support services and may also attract the interest of specialised professional bodies. The position of the speech therapist as both prop and stay and communication expert will be pointed out in relation to the different cases now about to be considered.

Acquired deafness
The professional workers to whom the patient may need access will include:
    Otologist
    Audiologist
    Teacher of the Deaf
    Hearing therapist
    Speech therapist.
The role of the speech therapist is to assist the patient to maintain his standard of speech. This is likely to become gradually eroded because of lack of auditory feedback. The first problems may occur in the regulation of voice quality, pitch and rate. Subsequently articulation may require attention.

Training foci
Representational system by which ideas may be received by lipreading. Re-training sound production hitherto monitored by ear; information must now be fed back through visual and tactile/proprioceptive pathways. Use of laryngograph or voiscope to retrain intonation. Use of other visual display systems operating in real time to show the person how to regulate speech and volume as well as pitch.

Training movement: Articulatory processes formerly under automatic regulation by the ear may now need to be brought more into conscious control and attention given to tactile and proprioceptive feedback.

Relaxation: This must be taught as a general state to prevent build up of anxiety but must also be directed to the vocal tract. Excessive tension here will restrict vocal function.

Auditory discrimination and judgement: Making use of a hearing aid; using overall redundancy to help interpret the message when acoustic information is insufficient.

Aphonia

The patient may lose his ability to produce voice because of surgery carried out to preserve life. The most extreme form is by total laryngectomy (for specialist literature in this field see bibliography).

The prognosis for learning to use pseudo-voice as an alternative to normal voice will depend upon the patient's health and the state of the pharyngeal tissue and muscles of respiration and articulation. Then all those aspects of morale, courage and buoyancy earlier touched upon will make a definitive difference. The level of communicative skill that can be achieved will depend also on the speaker's previous ability. If he had some experience of singing or public speaking his ear and respiration will be trained and he may articulate with clarity. The emotional colour of the normal voice depends upon flexible articulators and a relaxed pharynx. These are then orchestrated by the personality of the speaker and the style in which he places his emphasis or constructs his statements. This style will initially be lost and the patient concerned with the sheer mechanics of producing new sounds to convey meaning. As he becomes more proficient he will start to employ force and speed to make up for the absence of pitch. Even though he must reduce his phrase length he will learn to combine words skilfully so that his essential personality comes across. Speech therapists are often surprised by the individuality of expression, embracing dialect and occupation, which the laryngectomised person can command. To quote from an earlier work (1971) 'every speech therapist has her story to tell of the proficiency a laryngectomised patient can attain. We vie with each other in boasting of their attainments in using the telephone, in addressing business meetings, even in giving lectures.'

Professional workers involved will start with the ENT surgeon or otolaryngologist who has carried out the surgery and will include nurse, medical social worker and radiologist. The speech therapist will be responsible for teaching the patient how to speak again using either pseudo-voice or a vibrator. She will be greatly helped by former patients who have acquired such speech and who will visit the patient, demonstrate and encourage him. There are many associations for the laryngectomised and recently these have been brought together in Britain so that no laryngectomised patient need be without help.

Training Foci

Relaxation and Posture control: To induce ease and allow for most propitious placement and control of apparatus.

Respiratory modification: The patient's breathing is now independent of his 'voice' and must be disassociated in his mind also to prevent noisy over-blowing.

Sound production: Use of mechanical vibrator held against pharynx. Trapping of air in the pseudo-glottis and forcing it to vibrate (Snidecor, 1974). Use of carefully chosen consonants and vowels to assist trapping. Development of length of vibration.

Movement control: Co-ordination of 'voicing' with articulation.

Ear training: To allow for best standard of utterance in general and to lay the foundation for adequate monitoring.

Behaviour modification: To help the patient use his new voice effectively.

The rehabilitation of the laryngectomised patient through pseudo-voice is something of a special case in speech therapy. It involves teaching a compensatory method of utterance while yet encouraging the patient to present himself as speaking in the usual way. Other compensatory methods employ special apparatus or a special sign system. Here the patient uses speech which appears to accompany a vocal note. The note produced is therefore incongruous to those who believe the person to be speaking normally. It is deeper than the normal pitch except for a male bass and so women in particular tend to be conspicuous as soon as they start to speak. The treatment associated with the broad heading 'behaviour modification' is therefore of fundamental importance. The laryngectomised person must be helped to accept himself with his new voice if he is to stand up to the curiosity with which he may be regarded. An extremely positive approach must be adopted by the speech therapist and her demeanour during the early, difficult and messy stage of the first sounds may well determine how much the patient himself can accept.

The case of laryngectomy is the most extreme of the organic voice disorders and is included in this chapter because it focuses attention on the sudden deprivation which can afflict a normal speaker. The disease of cancer may of course attack other of the speech organs with consequent surgery leading to

Structural dysarthria

Rehabilatation in these cases would be the co-operative responsibility of the plastic surgeon, prosthetician and speech therapist who is concerned with communication.

She will therefore assist with the use of any prosthetic appliance and show the patient how to adapt his articulation to preserve intelligibility. An intelligent patient with good hearing will do much of the accommodation for himself but will need support.

The well regulated mechanics of utterance and highly developed language use stand a person in good stead if he has to undergo surgery for cancer of the tongue. Once more, this subject is one for the specialist but if an inexperienced speech therapist has to treat such a case she will find that the patient is able to use his speech memory, and this includes his phonetic memory to produce a sound which is acoustically acceptable. He may automatically substitute [f] or [v] for the now impossible [θ] and use the body and back of the tongue to manoeuvre the air stream for sibilants and fricatives. The speech therapist must help him to adopt these strategies if has not been able to find them for himself but she may find that the main part of her duties is to assist him to control his saliva and to eat in a manner acceptable to himself and others (for procedures for more radical conditions see Skelly, 1973).

We are again reminded that the speech apparatus is adapted from one that has the primary function of chewing and swallowing to maintain survival. The conditions giving rise to *neurological dysarthria* therefore will also cause difficulty with eating and control of saliva and these may have to be a first target in remediation. This speech disorder represents a mid-point between mechanical and linguistic disability since it occurs as the result of both subcortical and cortical lesions. In the latter cases it may be associated with language deficit and in the former with regulation of fluency (see Dalton and Hardcastle, op cit).

The speech therapist's first task is to carry out a comprehensive assessment of the dysarthric patient which will have as its basis the information given by the neurologist. If the patient has been referred from a general medical or geriatric ward there may be less precise information on neurological function than if he is in the care of a neurological or neurosurgical team. The speech therapist will hope to receive information as to the site and extent of the pathology and its effect upon function overall. She must then add her own detailed evaluation of the extent of the patient's communicative ability. The lesions may lie in the motor cortex of the cerebral hemispheres; in the pyramidal pathway or upper motor neurone; in the bulbar motor or lower motor neurones; in the basal ganglia; extra-pyramidal tracts and through the reticular formation to the cerebellar pathways; in the neuromuscular junction or the actual muscles themselves. Different syndromes will be produced as the result of the effect of the lesions on the complex innervatory system for respiration, phonation and articulation. The syndromes are described in standard neurological texts and for the purpose of this discussion three fairly standard conditions will be illustrated, those of bulbar palsy; pseudo-bulbar palsy; and Parkinson's disease.

As the incidence of acquired dysarthria is comparatively high it is surprising that so few speech therapists have looked for ways of assessing its effects. For many years the only real attempt at such assessement was that of Butfield (1961) and adaptations by her associates. A strong influence was later exerted on the British field by Darley (1975). Recently a new assessment has been devised by Enderby (1979) which offers British speech therapists an attractive alternative. Instead of using the medical categories and qualifying them as severe, moderate etc as has been the previous practise, Enderby suggests a profile of function in the areas of reflex activity; respiration; lips; jaw; palate; laryngeal and tongue. This is combined with an intelligibility rating and is to be taken together with a language assessment, medical information and some observations on the degree of insight, co-operation and motivation displayed by the patient. The speech therapist who has compiled her assessment may therefore look at the profile and see where she must start the rehabilitation process. This is in contrast to the results of medical type classification which suggest that strong differences in speech pattern are to be expected but which do not offer a lead into function and therefore the type of therapy to be selected.

Enderby's assessment also gives speech therapists opportunity to build up a collection of profiles which may be seen to be characteristic and which can therefore be used for teaching and research purposes. This once more shows the trend towards scientific handling of the data as our profession becomes more scholarly. We may hope to see the results of patients' progress being more accurately charted. The assessment given at different times with the three patients to be described would record the areas in which progress or deterioration was most marked as well as changing the rating on intelligibility.

Case 1: Mrs Black aged 62. The patient was first seen by the neurologist following her referral by her general practitioner. The complaint was of difficulty with swallowing and some slurring of speech. The diagnosis was of progressive bulbar palsy. The patient was not at first informed of this as the consultant neurologist considered that he knew too little about her as a person to assess how she could cope with such a pronouncement. The information was given to the G.P. and it was decided to inform Mrs Black's son. At some future date the patient was to be told, depending upon the progress of the disease. As Mrs Black had requested help with her speech, the referral was made with the request that the speech therapist did what she could to assist but did not inform the patient of the likely prognosis.

This position is an extremely difficult one for everybody and particularly for those in regular contact with the patient. In Mrs Black's case she accepted the statement of the neurologist that there had been some damage to the nerve supply which would interfere with normal speech. The immediate attitude shown by herself and supported by her son was to make the best of the position and try to speak intelligibly and without fatigue. There were therefore immediate therapy goals:

Focus of attention

Adapting rate of speech: It was necessary to teach phrasing and the use of pause so that more time could be given to articulation

Articulate speech practice: Breaking words into natural speech units or segments and improving articulatory placement

Maintaining voice quality: By working on strong yet smooth attack and practising phrases built round nasal consonants, open vowels and liquids to give resonance and ease.

There were also practical and moral considerations. If the speech therapist were to build up a close relationship with the patient it would be very difficult not to discuss prognosis. If she was to be dishonest with Mrs Black it would prevent her being able to give genuine human support when the true prognosis was discovered. It would also mean that the patient's confidence would be reduced over time as she became less able to maintain her speech. It would reasonably appear to her that speech therapy was not helpful and the therapist at best ineffective and at worst deceitful.

It was therefore decided to see Mrs Black twice a week for two weeks to work on the procedure listed. Then fortnightly treatments were established. These took the form of working sessions and advice. Thus rapport was maintained without too much discussion being invited. If questions such as 'will my speech really improve?' were asked they were answered 'your actual speech muscles are not going to get any stronger. We have to help you to speak in spite of this by doing slightly different things. What we are doing now seems to be helpful but if it stops being useful we will try something else'.

The opportunity to introduce the subject of non-verbal communication was sought and taken when the patient said 'it really is a terrible struggle to keep talking'. To this remark the therapist asked: 'Would you like to help yourself out by using some signing? It would be less tiring and your son and daughter-in-law can learn the signs too'. This was at first refused as had been expected. Mrs Black, an intelligent woman of fine character subsequently asked to see the neurologist again to discuss her condition. At that point he was able to tell her the true nature of the palsy. She then returned to the speech therapist for help in developing non-verbal communication.

Each patient is different, each situation is different and no general directive can really be given. The speech therapist has an early choice. She accepts the patient for help or she does not. Once accepted she must continue to do her best for him whether that involves speech rehabilitation, non-verbal communication, feeding assistance or family counselling.

Case 2: Mr White aged 69. This patient was referred by the geriatrician following several cerebro-vascular incidents which had resulted in bilateral damage to the pyramidal pathways. The condition was diagnosed as pseudo-bulbar palsy with consequent predominantly spastic dysarthria. As is common in such cases there was some evidence of damage other than upper motor neurone and the category might reasonably have been called 'mixed dysarthria'. The outstanding signs though were of spasticity with laboured, effortful movements of the articulatory organs.

Assesment revealed the following:

Reflexes: Sucking and jaw jerk reflexes were positive.

Respiration: Irregular. Adequate reciprocal action of respiratory muscles during quiet breathing but ill-co-ordinated in speech.

Lips: Poor closure at rest. Asymmetry with saliva escaping from right side. Alternate movements of rounding and relaxing, spreading and relaxing all attempted but performed very slowly. No lip shaping during speech; very weak labial plosives.

Jaw: Habitually held in the open position.

Palate: Patient can swallow fluids slowly. Eating is markedly slow but most foods attempted. Occasional dribbling. Some nasal contiguity of tone following nasal consonants.

Laryngeal: The sound 'ah' can be sustained for approximately 7 seconds with intermittent huskiness. Can produce notes of high and low pitch, but there is little pitch variation during speech. Volume is over-loud in speech. This can be controlled in short utterance.

Tongue: Normal appearance. Can protrude tongue well beyond lip margin but with asymmetrical movements; weakness on right side. Elevation performed slowly. Lateral movements slow and incomplete on left side. Alternate movements for 'ka-la' carried out very slowly and with effort.

Speech: Moderately intelligible for the most part. Articulatory detail is lost in continuous speech. Clusters are reduced. Patient finds continuous speech tiring and his performance deteriorates after a short time although he can continue to make himself understood.

Other information: Mr White is embarassed by ill-fitting dentures. He therefore tends to hold his head down which exascerbates difficulty in saliva control. He is somewhat labile but co-operative and fairly well motivated.

Language: Some word finding difficulty. Becomes confused if there are swift changes of subject.

Hearing: Mild to moderate loss in the high frequency range. Amplification not recommended yet.

Mr White was a good candidate for speech therapy and goals were easily established. An essential first step was to get a new set of dentures and this was done. Mr White's self respect and motivation for speech were considerably increased and he co-operated well in the following programme.

Training foci

1. All lip work was prefaced by jaw positioning first closed and then partly open. Lip closure, movement and control was started by the therapist gently pressing the patiet's lips together and requesting him to hold the position, followed by patient performing movement and attempting to increase pressure.
2. Strong and weak biting movements were contrasted. This was co-ordinated with swallowing. Followed by speaking aloud of plosive plus vowel combinations, e.g. 'bah, boo, boh.' Followed by words using these sounds placed in phrases with different stress. The same phrases were practised at reduced volume but

still maintaining stress patterns. Lingual consonants were then inserted after labials and nasals with intervening vowel, e.g. 'nobody' 'number one and number two' 'down the drain' and 'down the lane.'

3. Practice in chewing and swallowing was included in every session.

As the repertoire of clearly and strongly produced sounds in words increased Mr White was asked to concentrate on making the words distinctively different and thus started to take responsibility for monitoring his own speech. Additional therapy was provided to stimulate muscle tone by contrast stimulation. Tapping in the area of the cheeks and lips was carried out. Immediately following Mr White was asked to make a strong plosive sound 'b' and then a firm closure. Subsequently he was asked to produce labio-dentals with strong friction. This improved the sensation in the lip area.

The sounds 'ch' and 'sh' were practised with lip-rounded vowels 'chew', 'shoe', 'chop', 'shop', 'chore', 'shore'. These were placed in phrases and the phrases whispered with strong articulatory movement to induce co-articulation and more lip shaping in speech.

Back of tongue plosives were practised but with care in order to preserve the good phrase line. If the speech became broken up this area was temporarily abandoned and work on sustained vowels and phrasing reintroduced.

These specific tasks were followed by activities to improve overall intelligibility as control over short speech units improved. The activities included:

Training foci
Second stage:

Use of the telephone: This is important to maintain independence. Mr White practised saying his number and name and then gave short messages. He would telephone the speech therapist every week to confirm his appointment.

Narrative: Re-counting an incident or telling a short joke (most speech therapists agree that dysarthric patients should not be encouraged to tell long jokes).

At this stage general language practice was used to assist word finding and encourage conversational shift. It took the form of directed conversation with the therapist and some word games, e.g. animal, vegetable or mineral which depend upon asking questions. These could be played at home with Mr White's grandchildren. Measures to involve the family were always taken so long as they were compatible with Mr White's self respect. Mr White was then required to make word lists for himself beginning with different sounds and practise them routinely as a limbering up exercise. He was also asked to define words in the speech clinic and to produce synonyms. These provided variety and also meant that he improved his ability to assist himself out of a difficulty if his articulation let him down.

Mrs White did not attend every session with her husband. This was not considered necessary after the first few sessions. He was strong enough to travel on his own by hospital transport and it was considered that he should take responsibility for his own progress. Contact with the speech therapist was maintained by telephone calls which Mrs White or her daughters initiated. Treatment on a regular basis was terminated when Mr White was able to maintain intelligibility and control in ordinary conversation but regular review was carried out.

This case shows a comparatively straightforward rehabilitation job where the mechanics of speech have let the patient down but where he has retained reasonably good ability to co-operate in treatment and where no strongly adverse psychological factors are operating. The important elements to emphasise are:

Practical and useful rehabilitation procedures

Letting the patient carry as much responsibility as he can.

The third case showed the patient to a large extent taking the lead in his therapy.

Case 3: Dr Green aged 65 observed in himself the first signs of Parkinson's disease. He was a gynaecologist so he sought confirmation from a neurologist colleague. Upon receiving it he requested an appointment with the speech therapist so that he could learn how to maintain his speech for as long as possible. He wished to continue in practice so long as his tremor did not place any patient at risk. He also hoped to be able to speak in public about childbirth and child rearing and to write on the subject. He therefore hoped to use a dictaphone or dictate to his secretary.

In addition to his professional work Dr Green had a very wide circle of friends with whom he hoped to keep in touch. He was therefore extremely well motivated to maintain his speech while yet realising the prognosis.

The speech therapist is a privileged person in that she is allowed to meet and work with people of Dr Green's calibre who come to her for help but from whom she cannot fail to learn. But her responsibility to such people is very great. They are prepared to make strong demands on themselves so she must also give them the best advice possible and be quite sure that she is thoroughly up to date in all that she recommends.

Procedure: The nature of Parkinson's disease and its effects on speech were discussed in detail. Dr Green resembled many medical specialists in knowing a great deal about his own subject but not very much about speech. He was therefore genuinely interested to learn how the vocal note is monitored and to take part in laboratory investigations to show vocal cord activity. He also learned to study spectographs intelligently and to use a sound level meter in vocal regulation. The voiscope was not at that time available but it would be an ideal instrument for such a patient.

Assessment: A characteristic picture of mild Parkinsonian dysarthria was revealed. Lip and facial muscles were slightly stiff giving the start of the characteristic mask-like expression of the disease. Dr Green wished to maintain facial expression so far as he could because he realised the effect on his patients of any failure of responsiveness by him.

Training focus
First stage:
Conscious work to improve sensation associated with smiling, frowning, and looking questioningly. As the muscles around the eyes were less affected than those of the face and lips it was found that expression could be induced by working on different kinds of regard – wrinkling of the forehead, raising of the eyebrows contrasted with straight gaze. Imitation of the therapist was only used occasionally for fear of introducing artificiality. It was considered more important to underline Dr Green's own manner but to assist him to combine those elements – warm strong tone and straight regard – which could reassure others.

Assessment further revealed the start of the festinating utterance by which the patient becomes less and less intelligible with increased speed. So the above procedures were combined with short statements – don't worry' and 'take a deep breath' – Dr Green learned not to combine too many instructions on one breath himself. He also carried out regular practice to maintain clear articulation.
Second stage:
Phrasing and control of length. Instructions were given with different emphasis but with attention to natural rhythm. Dr Green was encouraged to start using a dictaphone and to work out a sensible length of utterance which he could maintain. He was then asked to dictate in this manner to his secretary. Dr Green practised putting

several prepared passages together and giving short lectures to the therapist on easy childbirth or some such useful topic on which he was an authority. His audience was then increased by adding speech therapy students.

Gradually it became apparent that the laryngeal area was going to prove the major handicap. Talks to midwives and prospective mothers were therefore pre-recorded and given, amplified, with Dr Green attending the gathering to answer questions. A voice microphone or laryngeal amplifier was made for him by the hospital physics laboratory and this was very helpful (see Allan, 1970).

Third stage:

Preserving vocal strength. Voice exercises were started by slight pressure of the hands against each other associated with glottal closure (Butfield, 1961) and this followed by voicing. Dr Green was then asked to repeat the same sounds without the initial pushing exercise. The voice amplifier was introduced. Dr Green also practised with the sound level meter and by talking into a candle flame. This relatively mundane device is helpful in that if too much breath is released the flame wavers but if full voicing is used it stays constant. It can still be recommended to those (many) who lack sophisticated electronic or mechanical apparatus.

By such means as these, explained and buttressed by discussion, Dr Green maintained his communication power for the maximum time and inspired the speech therapist to the highest level of ingenuity of which she was capable in order to keep up with him. It should be remembered that it is the patient's own goals that are important and the speech therapist should only seek to lower them if they are patently unrealistic and their pursuit leading to frustration and depression. With patients of high ability, honesty and insight, the speech therapist should not content herself by offering a reduced goal on the grounds that it is reasonable for the majority (Lott, 1979).

Skinner recommends group work for those Parkinson's patients who are less highly motivated as regular practice is so important. This practice can be carried out helpfully where a certain amount of competition is available. All dysarthric patients need work on the mechanics of speech and regular exercise and repetition are essential. The purpose of the group is not for social support, though this can be a side product, but to allow drills to be carried out with the most economical use of therapist's time and minimum of tedium for the patient. Patients, such as Mr White may be enrolled also in Stroke clubs which are intended chiefly for social support. Some of these clubs have been started by speech therapists whose patients lack motivation to communicate because their lives are so passive, restricted or isolated. Or the speech therapist may refer patients to groups run by volunteers such as those organised by the Chest and Heart Association. These groups arose following the impetus given by Valerie Eaton Griffith's work with aphasic people in making members of the community take responsibility for improving communication in the handicapped.

Aphasia

The condition of aphasia is one which attracts many professional workers as well as volunteers. Here the patient has lost control over his ability to convey and receive ideas or even basic information through the medium of language. He needs the services of two groups of people. Those who try to restore him to some place in society and those who wish to find out more about the processes of language and thought by studying the manner in which elements have been lost and retained. In the first category we may place:
Medical rehabilitation team
The social worker
The marriage guidance counsellor
The re-settlement officer
The volunteer.
and most prominently among the second group:
The linguist
The psychologist.
This is not to imply that the two last named professions may not be extremely helpful to the patient in devising methods which aid recovery. However, it is not usual for them to work on a regular basis with a large number of adults with acquired aphasia. Nor is it to suggest that the first group of workers lack intellectual curiosity, but their task is to provide the greatest good for the greatest number. The speech therapist can be seen as linking the groups and she belongs to each. She has a strong service commitment to all aphasic patients who need help at any level and must therefore be practical in what she undertakes to do for them. She is also continually and fundamentally concerned with how language works and thence how it can be made to function. So she will ally herself with those who are trying to improve the patient's function and restore him to society and she will turn to those who can offer her more insight into the exact nature of the patients's disability.

In the case of Mr B. (Chapter 3) some 10 professional workers assisted him at various times during his years of rehabilitation but the speech therapist was the continuing link. It was her job to think of ways by which the best use could be made of research findings to stimulate verbal comprehension, and word retrieval, and also to try to keep the patient going during periods of ill-health and depression. It was her task to beat any circumstance which threatened to overwhelm her patient into a series of miniscule tasks which he could deal with. The circumstance might be:

Telephoning
Map reading
Following the news on television
Stocking up his garden
Buying a birthday present for his wife
Booking a table in a restaurant
Consulting a railway timetable
Making an appointment to see his doctor.

Speech therapy for aphasic adults is not given with the naive idea of teaching the patient to speak as he did before. It is given to help him go on with his life; a life which had been pervaded by speech and which must now be re-created using the fragments, or the major corpus that remains.

In order to do her job effectively the speech therapist must have some model of the patient's language to work on. Hence the development of very detailed tests for aphasia and the exposition of theoretical models which engender them.

A first object of tests for aphasia is to distinguish that state from dysarthria or apraxia.

Dysarthria
The speech disorders result from disturbances in muscle control over the speech mechanism. The pattern of movement tends to be constant and the limitations may be systematically charted.

Apraxia
The disorder arises from impairment in the capacity to position and regulate the muscles and to carry out a learned sequence of movements. The resulting patterns of movement and therefore speech are inconsistent and not always predictable from an assessment based either on motor or linguistic analysis. Assessment must also concern itself with the whole movement schema which underlies the activity.

A/dysphasia
The disorder is rooted in the impairment of language functioning. Assessment of the functioning, if carried out when the patient's

condition has been stabilised should provide a picture of assets and liabilities which may guide the therapist in her rehabilitation programme.

If cerebral damage is extensive these conditions may occur together.

So we may find:

Dysarthria plus apraxia

Here the patient has consistent limitations on the movements of his articulators in both speech and non speech function. He has considerably more difficulty in positioning for speech than the movement limitations suggest.

Therapeutic focus: Must therefore be upon improving movement awareness. Passive manipulation followed by passive-assisted movement then active imitation should be attempted. P.N.F. procedures (Langley and Darvill, 1979) may be used to advantage. The patient has a memory of the target sound and this should be used immediately following the stimulative procedures. Automatic and highly overlearned speech, e.g. counting should be used. As the mechanism starts to function word lists should be practised starting with nasals and glides and working up to plosives. Affricates and fricatives will be particularly difficult.

The aim should be for intelligible utterance accepting that this may have to be slow and sparse.

Dysarthria plus aphasia

The co-existence of a severe dysarthric element will force the decision as to whether speech is a realistic goal. If the aphasia is mild and the patient possesses moderately good comprehension, speech rehabilitation should be attempted. If there is very poor comprehension with inability to control jargon and cease unintelligible utterance, speech stimulation should not be given. Instead of one overriding aim, there must be several specific ones.

Therapeutic foci:
1. Improvement of chewing, swallowing and general feeding and self care
2. Comprehension training
3. Re-education in writing.

Response to these will indicate whether spoken language may be tackled

Apraxia plus aphasia

In order to determine whether there is co-existence of apraxia and aphasia and the consequent prognosis for therapy one must look more searchingly at the models underlying assessment. If apraxia is present it tends to dominate considerations of treatment since an apraxic patient will not improve unless he speaks. He should not however be stimulated to speak if his comprehension deficit is severe (see p. 226). We must first explore the control the patient can exert at an inhibitory level. If inhibition is present some volitional activity may be hoped for.

We cannot therefore escape considerations of neurological organisational hierarchies when considering volitional language behaviour. Such considerations have dominated the thinking of some researchers into aphasia. (Luria, 1966 and 1970). Students starting to work in the field of aphasia must first revise their neurophysiology and neuropathology to appreciate the contribution of Luria and of Geschwind (among others). They must then look at psychological models to appreciate the contributions of Wepman (1961) and Porch (1967). They are then recommended to read Lesser's valuable text on linguistic investigations of aphasia (1978). In studying the individual aphasic we are looking at a damaged version of a once intact and highly elaborate language organisation. The individual quality of the original performance has already been pointed out, but mechanisms and functions in individuals are subject to the same stresses and tend to break down in similar ways. It is because patterns of breakdown are similar that assessments can be used across broad groups. It is because individual need differs that rehabilitation programmes must be individually constructed.

The first published test for aphasia by a speech therapist in this country is that of Butfield (1952). Individual tests were developed subsequently by a number of British therapists such as Fawcus M. and Hatfield who were interested in the subject and in teaching it to students. None of these tests were standardised and succeeding assessments were based on American models. The reason was a simple one and concerned the training of speech therapists and their lack of access to measurement and statistical techniques. Unfortunately this has lead to some distrust of aphasia assessments by clinicians who have worked for a long time without them and feel them to be excessively time consuming in relation to the information yielded. The new generation of speech therapists is taking to such assessments very naturally but is sometimes at a loss as to how to proceed without them. The purpose of testing aphasic patients was stated by the Boston team of Goodglass and Kaplan (1976) to be '1. Diagnosis of presence and type of aphasic syndrome, leading to inferences concerning cerebral localisation

2. measurement of the level of performance over a wide range, for both initial determination and detection of change over time; comprehensive assessment of the assets and liabilities of the patient in all language areas as a guide to therapy'.

This fairly represents the aims of most of the tests in common use though some incline more towards the measurement of abilities and others toward the therapeutic guide. The thoroughness with which they explore the whole language process also varies. Some assessments are frankly designed as screening procedures and do not purport to examine abilities in depth. The speech therapist must therefore be selective and know why she is carrying out the assessment and what she hopes to gain from it. The areas of investigation are clearly stated in all standardised tests. If the speech therapist considers that these are not likely to be sufficiently searching in one or other area she should consult the psychologist who may be able to offer further ways of looking at cognitive function with regard to language. She should also make use of linguistic analysis and seek help from linguists in probing out the areas of deficit in high level patients for whom standardised assessments are rarely sufficiently searching. Reference has already been made to the case of Mr B. and here the contributions of the psychologist and linguist in throwing light on the way in which the patient handled language was invaluable (Byers Brown and Ives, 1969 and Cruse, 1978). Such contributions assist the speech therapist particularly in the area of recall and cueing which form such a high percentage of her work in aphasia. The student therapist is therefore recommended to go beyond the material on aphasia offered in texts of speech pathology and learn in her student days to seek help from research findings in neuropsychology and psycholinguistics (Hatfield, 1972). It is only by such methods that we will extend the therapy techniques which have been constant for too long (for summary of such techniques see Halpern, 1972).

The position in aphasia is at present an interesting one. Older practitioners (including this author) who have worked with many aphasic patients are in no doubt that speech therapy is helpful. They have records, letters and memories to prove how much individual families have valued their care. But now that speech therapists. are asking for more responsibility and increased numbers (Quirk, 1972) they are required to be accountable. This accountability is not, as was pointed out by Darley (1972) demanded in all branches of healing. 'Much that goes on in psychiatry, physical medicine, neurology and other medical fields has not been subjected to the kind of rigorous evaluation discussed here, but patients come to these specialists for treatment and they get it.' So there is no need for the speech therapy profession to become excessively anxious or to castigate itself unduly. There is every need for it to be clear and realistic as to what it can accomplish. It has repeatedly been stated that a speech therapist should not be employed if someone else can do the job better. It is now possible for speech therapists and volunteers to work together and this would seem excellent for those many patients who need considerable help but whose general condition and prognosis does not justify intensive professional therapy. Several research projects are under way to assess the relative roles of professional and volunteer workers. Such studies need to be rigorously drawn up or they will generate false conclusions which will feed prejudice and parsimony.

The speech therapist working with aphasic patients is first reminded that she must do so in propitious circumstances if she is to help him. This means that she consider:

1. Medical and professional arguments as to the nature and timing of intervention (see bibiliography).
2. The physical and geographical conditions in which speech therapy is carried out (see Chapter 4).

The author in a very early study (Fitch, 1957) looked at adult aphasic patients who received bi-weekly speech therapy as outpatients at a large general hospital. The value of speech therapy was stated as lying in 'the stimulus it gives the patient to communicate; the insight it helps him to develop into his condition and the extent to which it can help him to come to terms with his environment. The patient's needs were seen to be:

To re-establish communication, at first by whatever means he can

To be helped to understand the nature of his difficulties so that he may work to overcome them

To be protected from the demands of relatives, friends and associates who cannot appreciate his condition and may therefore be perpetually provoking situations leading to failure and frustration. Later the patient must be helped to come to terms with these demands.

Speech therapy directed towards meeting these needs would be most efficacious if given where:

1. The patient's efforts to communicate are appreciated
2. There is concurrent treatment for associated handicaps
3. The environment is adjusted so that no excessive demands are made on the patient.

Such conditions may be found in a rehabilitation centre where there is a team of workers including physiotherapists, medical gymnasts, occupational therapists and speech therapists under the direction of a specialist in rehabilitation and under the guidance of the neurologist and psychologist. Full co-operation between members of such a team should be of maximum assistance in helping the patient to regain as much as possible of his lost function. The patient may also receive a large measure of support from working with a congenial group where he will find company, recreation and stimulus.'

It is sad to record that there has been little growth in the number of rehabilitation centres developed since that was written and that there is so little chance of their number being considerably increased in the near future. Even if they were to be increased there would still be many aphasic patients who would not be able to benefit from them. Such establishments are expensive and must accordingly be selective. They must by definition exclude the elderly and sick for whom an intensive, generalised programme of rehabilitation is not indicated. Any speech therapist can see the justification for this exclusion and will therefore be prepared to seek the help of the geriatrician and stroke club organiser in providing additional and ongoing support for such patients. But another group to be excluded is that of the aphasic patient whose additional handicaps are not sufficiently severe to merit total rehabilitation in a multi-disciplinary centre. This almost certainly includes the patient with a temporal or parietal lesion which does not cause severe hemiplegia. Yet these patients are among the most tragically isolated and the most in need of support because they cannot handle incoming messages nor conduct themselves in a speaking society. It was the author's long experience with patients of this nature, rendered excessively dependent upon the speech therapist as their sole ally (see anecdotal account, 1971) which has convinced her of the need for a more total approach to any kind of rehabilitation for aphasia. In the cited study these patients were considered very carefully in the effort to see whether the routine provision of bi-weekly out-patient speech therapy could in any way meet their needs.

'This is the group that constitutes the speech therapist's greatest responsibility. Speech therapy may have to be a lifeline to them, linking their activities and occupying their time. The speech therapist must be prepared to spend a considerable amount of time, probably outside clinic hours, giving support and guidance in all sorts of situations because she is the only person the patient has who comes anywhere near understanding what his condition is doing to his life.

The speech therapist must explore all the speech and language situations which the patient may be confronted with in order to find effective and helpful ways of dealing with them. These situations will vary according to the patient's domestic situation but may include: time telling, asking for bus fares, calculating change, shopping, telephoning, reading the newspaper and playing cards as well as conversation. Specific techniques must be devised in the clinic which may be reinforced in the environment. — It is up to the speech therapist to devise and if necessary to create situations in which they may be reinforced.'

Looking at the present day position it may be stated that the speech therapist should use her clinical time to explore and introduce methods which will assist communicative recovery and involve other people in creating a matrix of support within which the recovery may be accelerated. It is the continuing practice of bringing severely handicapped patients to hospital out-patient clinics; involving hospital transport with all its vagaries and fatigues; exposing the patient to inevitable delay and heightening his anxiety by the process which renders him almost inaccessible to rehabilitation. Yet it is within these conditions in Britain that speech therapy is still judged. The findings generated in the U.S. on methods and recovery rates are where therapy is intensive and working conditions good. One U.S. study where the patients were not carefully selected and were given only 40 hours therapy showed no gains as the result of this. The study (Sarno, Silverman and Sands, 1970) has frequently been quoted to show that speech therapy is not generally effective in Britain. A more proper conclusion would be that the way in which speech therapy is administered in most health areas makes it almost impossible for the patient to realise his recovery potential and places a heavy burden on the therapist who has to compensate by her own exertions for so many deficiencies in the system.

Now in order to be fair it must also be said that deficiencies in the conditions in which speech therapy is given must not be offered as excuses for the lack of resource and imagination which are all too frequently encountered. The proper use of assessment, stimulatory techniques, re-training, experiment and environmental support may at present be seen as the way to approach therapy for aphasic patients. While all the procedures overlap to some extent the timing will be dictated by the patient's state. In the 1957 study it was found that there were three phases of treatment which varied in length but which were distinctive and need different approaches and material. These related to:

1. Period of emotional shock and instability: It was suggested that treatment during this stage should make use of general material which was familiar but neutral. Emphasis on family or personal matters which would show up the present state too acutely was to be avoided
2. Period of rediscovery: As some recovery occurs or as the patient becomes more stable, material directly related to the patient's life should be used to revive associations
3. Period of consolidation or redirection: Depending upon the prognosis it may be necessary for the patient to work hard to recover special abilities or to turn his thoughts to other outlets and activities.

The two early stages may be deemed to occur within the period of spontaneous recovery which most authorities suggest may continue until about 6 months after the episode with the most dramatic changes happening early. Both research evidence and individual testimony now suggest that recovery can go on occurring after the first year. The contribution of therapy has usually been seen as most conspicuously demonstrated when spontaneous recovery has slowed down. We would be better advised to concentrate more attention on the early stages and assist spontaneous recovery. This would give impetus to continuing work by the patient and might give a better overall result. However, it is probably necessary to rely on stimulation rather than the use of compensatory techniques until it becomes clear that the patient has failed to revive effective strategies.

Case histories cited in the British Journal or the Bulletin of the College of Speech Therapists support the idea that a change of technique or new approach will be required sometime after the first year of therapy. This may be because the patient has arrived at a plateau or because reassessment has suggested something new. Sometimes the fresh approach is hailed as a much more effective method when it is only its timing that has produced the change. Both the patient and the therapist needed another impetus. The reason for the improvement is important for research purposes but is of less importance to the therapist and particularly to the patient and his family than the fact that it has occurred. What is essential is that the speech therapy team can continue to offer fresh appraisals and ideas which are well indicated by continuing investigation and are not random. In a very handicapped patient the process could be:

Phase 1: Patient is seen on the ward. Preliminary screening shows global aphasia affecting all modalities. The speech therapist visits the patient regularly and guides the ward staff as to how to speak to him and what to demand. She gives the patient a communication chart and instructs him, his family and ward staff in its use.

Phase 2: Patient leaves hospital and is seen as an out-patient. His wife accompanies him. The first sessions are spent in exploring the patient's ability and showing his wife how to get non-verbal responses rather than pressing for speech. The patient uses a few automatic utterances. Comprehension appears very limited. Further testing is postponed. Graded auditory stimulation is given with patient being required to listen and identify.

Phase 3: After three months the patient is showing improved comprehension and can identify objects and pictures. He can obey a two part command. He now possesses some automatic speech, e.g. counting, yes and no. He can repeat wife's name.

At this point the speech therapist is actively planning support for the patient. He is not moving in such a way as to suggest that communication is going to be regained without a long period of work. A group or stroke club should be sought. This will take some of the onus of help from the patient's wife and give him something to contribute. The speech therapist will probably move into more active therapy using word repition and sentence completion techniques. She will administer a full scale aphasia assessment or as much of it as the patient can manage and will use it as a baseline for progress measurement.

Phase 4: The patient's attendance and progress could be:

Attended as an out-patient for about a year. His attendances varied but averaged about twice weekly

OR

The patient has been seen three times a week for six months and then given a break as no significant progress was being made

OR

The patient was not given individual therapy following his admission to a speech club but the active therapy suggested was carried out by the group which met twice weekly. When reassessed by the speech therapist the patient showed considerable gains in speech as judged by length of utterance, speed, accuracy of repetition and the variety of linguistic forms employed

OR

The patient has made steady and sustained progress in individual therapy given twice weekly. Progress was judged as above and could also be recorded on the test for aphasia.

Thus do speech therapist and patient arrive at points of decision. Depending on what has been done and how the patient has responded the therapist may:

Request a further neurological or other medical examination

Propose that some system of non-verbal communication, e.g. Bliss be used

Set up a series of counselling sessions for the family

Establish a clearly defined and linguistically based programme to consolidate and expand syntax

Devise a cueing programme to facilitate word recall

Put the patient on to a system of programmed instruction

Abandon specific therapy and develop general techniques of discussion and stimulation to help patient develop his own insight into what is going on.

Such decisions are neither arbitrary nor whimsical. They are arrived at by two people as the result of what is happening to one of them and what resources are available to the other. They reveal the kind of thinking and planning which goes on in the speech clinics and which are frequently summarised as 'conventional speech therapy.'

The speech therapist may use published, standardised assessments to cut down on some of the decisions she needs to make. If, on testing by the Minnesota Test for Differential Diagnosis (Schuell, 1964) at around six months post-stroke, the patient is revealed as having 'irreversible aphasic syndrome characterised by almost complete loss of language skills' there would be little point in continuing individual therapy. If he was revealed on the Boston assessment as a case of severe Broca's aphasia the thrust of therapy must continue to be devoted towards verbal production and imitation techniques. Melodic intonation therapy (Sparks et al, 1974) and syntax training may be used, or the speech therapist may use the standardised tests as a guide to progress. She may carry out her assessment, using a technique devised for a particular purpose — multi-sensory cueing, delayed imitation – and then repeat her assessment or the relevant section after a couple of months to see what gains had been made. Again she may make her own linguistic analysis, recording class and number of verbal structures attempted by the patient and repeating the analysis at intervals after training. The important thing is to formulate some aim and have a means of checking how that aim is being reached. It is bad for everyone concerned to let speech therapy continue at infrequent intervals but over a long period of time for vague purposes of 'morale' or in the hope of a positive change of state without any indication as to what could promote it.

Much of what the therapist does can be quantified, but there have been no attempts to consider the therapist's own speech or input as a factor in her patients progress. Such an evaluation would be very difficult. However, it might show that the range of language used by the therapist had a definite relationship to that used by the patient. Or, the speech therapist is using herself more than the material she selects to get the required results. This statement invites the corollary that some speech therapists use their own input more skilfully than do others and rely upon it more.

When the patient's language is affected only at a high level the speech therapist will have to use her own language skills to an even greater extent. The material on which they both work will be that which allows memory, verbal judgements, discrimination and reasoning to be re-trained. There will be no packaged material ready to hand so the therapist will use guided discussion as one of her chief methods of stimulation. This may be supported by subsequent work with the tape recorder and by reading and precis and dictation. But the onus will still be on the medium of verbal exchange to provide motivation and stimulate insight. The speech therapist should not discharge the high level dysphasic, any more than the dysarthric, until she has helped him to reach a level of function where he feels secure and relaxed and able to pursue his own way of life.

The tendency to refer to the speech therapist only the severely aphasic patient because the better ones will manage somehow is an unfortunate one. It deprives both patient and therapist of the chance to polish up their language skills and to gain additional insight into the condition of dysphasia. We all learn a great deal from our intellectually demanding patients and we need to work with them for their sakes and for our own.

12

The position re-stated

A great deal of the work described reveals the speech therapist in her established role. She works on an individual basis as a clinician moving from medical knowledge to educative application. She represents a caring profession with its own discipline. The effectiveness of her therapy is rooted in knowledge of normal and pathological conditions and in her sharing of the human predicament. In order to maintain and develop this classic role speech therapy students will need a broadly based undergraduate course of study which proceeds to specialisation in the final years.

The College of Speech Therapists has been under some pressure to consider limited qualifications which would entitle the graduate to work only with children or only with adults. This it has steadfastly refused to do. Its attitude is supported by the Department of Health and Social Security. The Committee of Enquiry recommended that speech therapy be unified under health instead of the previous division into education and health. This unification, which has been implemented, means that both children and adults can be treated at any speech clinic in the area.

Although the service will naturally develop sites and accommodation suitable for particular clinical populations, there is no bar to a patient receiving treatment because the therapist works for a different authority.

It is extremely important for a small body of colleagues such as speech therapists to be able to make the utmost of their combined resources whether these lie in specialist knowledge, equipment or accommodation. It is also very much better for morale for young speech therapists to be in regular touch with each other as well as having the benefit of discussion with more senior colleagues. The newly qualified will have recently emerged from several years of student life where the sharing of ideas was a constant feature. While they are now equipped to work independently, they need to continue to receive the kind of stimulation which will not only help their immediate therapy but will lead them to produce new methods of treatment and management.

As the move towards an integrated service has gathered momentum, speech therapists have needed to refresh their knowledge of treatment methods for those populations previously served elsewhere. Training speech therapists in an initial general competence will not obviate the need for refresher courses since no person can keep up to-date without help and stimulation. But, of course, no person can keep abreast of advances in all fields. The integrated service depends on specialists within its ranks who can take responsibility for certain conditions. By developing special expertise they act as resource people for the rest of the team.

It is common for students to be attracted to particular handicaps during their training, or even to become interested in speech therapy because of early acquaintance with a particular condition, but it is unwise to encourage too early or too intensive a specialisation. Many students who believe that they will be happiest working with children begin to enjoy the stimulation offered by adult patients as they themselves become more competent and mature. Also, speech therapy students who feel at a loss during their first essays into pre-school work may later find themselves accommodating with ease and pleasure to the demands of young children. The comfort that the student experiences in working with different cases is, of course, highly dependent on her understanding of their condition and what she believes she has to offer.

It has already been pointed out that students of speech therapy have many sources of information. We are indeed approaching the position of medicine where students have too large a mass of factual information to be able to handle it and too limited clinical exposure to learn by experience. Teaching must then emphasise principles and seek to make them understood. Information must be correlated across subjects and between lecture theatre and clinic. The student can help considerably in her own education by working actively to achieve this. Such an attitude will stand her in very good stead as she moves into clinical practice. The whole field, as may be seen from the foregoing chapters, is burgeoning and there are no areas where we can feel that all the important questions have been answered, or even been asked. Many areas would repay the fresh application of psychology and as the explicit contribution of this subject has been rather neglected in these pages it will be considered a little more here. It has been implicitly recognised in all those aspects of therapist-patient care which penetrate beneath the straightforward surface relationship. As was stated in Chapter 3 the psychologist has always been called upon by the speech therapist to guide her through the complexities of human behaviour but the insightful penetration of human behaviour is only one aspect of psychology. The psychologist has become much more active and not only observes and interprets behaviour but takes the lead in shaping it. He not only assesses a person's intellectual skills but seeks to develop them.

Broadbent (1971) commenting on the large and expanding field of cognitive psychology represented by a selection of its papers states that psychology has 'reached a point where it can usefully tackle many problems nearer to ordinary human concerns than were the problems of traditional psychophysics or conditioning.' The author, reviewing the same work comments that 'speech therapists are certainly among those immersed in human concerns, indeed frequently submerged by them. The practising clinician is rarely able to isolate the primary disabilities of the language disordered from the consequent social and behavioural problems imposed. The necessity to be concerned in general management can lead to diminuition of the drive to understand the primary condition.' In recommending the papers, the point is also made that the 'attention focused upon the relationship between language skills and conceptual thinking is most valuable for a profession which is necessarily concerned with verbal detail.'

We are surely due for an extension of our clinical methods as the result of the application of cognitive psychology. Very few of these are at present based upon stimulating the patient's thinking as a route to language. This is perhaps surprising in view of the lip service long paid to Piaget, whose work figures prominently on every psychology syllabus for speech therapy students. We have made very little use in our clinical work of the directive aspect of speech and the way speech is used by children to organise their behaviour. This is also surprising in view of the interest which greeted the experiments and hypotheses of Luria in the late 1950s and the present day emphasis on attention training and other routes towards individual organisation. While much time is spent in speech clinics teaching form and structure and also in stimulating a flow of speech, it is not often that even such simple activities as those following are employed.

Case report: Alan aged 6 years.
Background information: slow to acquire speech but was not referred for speech therapy. Does not show any phonological impairment but his teacher notes a lack of verbal ease together with some adjustment problems. When assessed by the psychologist he

showed poor vocabulary development and poor verbal reasoning together with rigidity in many aspects of behaviour. Alan and the therapist work together at a table separated from each other by a cardboard screen which hides each section from the other. They then take it in turns to give each other directions using their own material.

Therapist: I'm putting my red house next to the little bridge. You do the same thing.' (Child complies) 'Let's see if our sides look the same – yes, they do, good.'

Alan: 'I'm putting my house near the tree.'

When they check they find that the therapist using the same man-oeuvre had put her red house beside a large tree whereas Alan had put his yellow house in front of a small tree. Neither was wrong but more exactitude was required. As the game continues commands become more accurate and the next stage can be tried.

Therapist: 'I want to get my car across the bridge but I can't do it' (their toys are identically arranged).

Alan: 'Go straight down the road.'

Therapist: 'But I've banged into the tree.'

Alan: 'Go down the road and stop.'

Therapist: 'Stop before I get to the tree?'

Alan: 'Yes.'

Therapist: 'Right. Now what shall I do?'

Alan: 'You can go across the bridge now.'

This type of activity helps to develop some exactitude and some realisation as to the importance of words to convey ideas. It can be used with many language impaired and disordered children. So can the following. Therapist and child put out a set of cards, the famil-iar sequencing material now very popular in the speech clinic.

Therapist: 'Tell me about these pictures' (they have arranged them in sequence).

Alan: 'The cat is looking at the fish. The cat is getting on the table. The cat is putting his arm into the fish tank. The fish tank is broken.'

Therapist: 'And where is the fish?'

Alan: 'The cat has eat the fish up.'

Therapist: 'Now tell me the story as if you were the fish.'

Alan: 'I am swimming in my tank. The cat is coming in. The cat is getting on the table. The cat is eating me up.'

Therapist: 'Now tell me the story as if you were the cat.'

These activities show the start of imaginative and also precise activities which children must employ if they are to move freely in language. The work of Vygotsky and Luria could stimulate many more activities of this nature using the directing and modifying functions of language. Therapists who are used to working in this way will move more happily into the cognitive linguistic field opened up by Bates (1976) than will those who see their therapeutic role as one concentrated upon language form. Other therapists may seek help from Halliday (1975) in developing a functional-interactive approach. They may learn to appraise verbal activity not just as to whether it is clear and correct in form but whether it is successful in conveying the message economically and without ambiguity.

The plight of an adult patient with acquired dysphasia deserves attention here. He has presumably been able to understand how language functions, but he may well be reduced to concretism rather than able to use abstraction in his thinking and this may interfere with his understanding of verbal messages. The therapist must take care not to confuse even when she believes herself to be assisting comprehension. She needs help from linguists and psychologists to set up experiments which will show the level at which the patient can co-operate in language exchange. Results of the experiments will suggest the way in which to stimulate his own thought word processes. There is a rich field of therapeutic techniques to be developed as our understanding of language use and language function matches up to our understanding of its form. These techniques have hardly been touched upon in present methods aimed at stimulating the verbal processes of adult aphasic patients. As it is, most of their speech work is ego-centred and can contribute to the passivity so often encountered in the brain damaged adult. A great deal of the material used in group work for aphasics is based upon simple turn taking and stimulus response. It would be helpful to many if more active contributions were required through the need to direct each other. As electronic devices become cheaper and more plentiful, suitable adult toys may be devised which need explicit instructions before yielding responses – a kind of verbal fruit machine in fact. The line joining an ingenious device and a basic cognitive skill must be drawn by the therapist but she will certainly find her colleagues in psychology a great source of help.

When the new generation of speech therapists starts to exert major influence upon its profession it may be more in the direction to which many psychologists are tending. Instead of adhering as closely as their predecessors to the position of the clinical guru, they may move more strongly towards that of social explorer. Many of the conditions presented in Chapters 7 and 8 may not be treated clinically but tackled socially. There will be much more interest in the way in which people use language and need to use it; also as to how the attitudes of others impinge upon these needs. Children failing to conform to normal language criteria may be examined as much in the playground as in clinic to find the blocking elements. The therapist in clinic may be deemed to know far too little about the contexts that most motivate speech and so she may find herself moving into the community in order to find out more and thus influence more. This has happened in stammering where the tension between speaker and group has always been seen as profoundly important. The speech therapist should certainly not fear such a move as diluting her own contribution. It will give her new ways in which to make use of her techniques of analysis and remediation but with perhaps more realisation of the communicative cosmos.

Speech therapists have not yet paid much heed to the concept of the 'speech act' or to the principles which speakers must follow in order to keep a conversation going. We are perhaps too used to carrying the communicative burden and encouraging participation by reassuring support rather than by tacit requirement. We have not yet made sufficiently clear analyses of our own verbal behaviour to see whether we do really help our patients to appreciate or relearn the conversational principle. It is particularly necessary for those therapists who place great emphasis upon their own speech as therapeutic agent (see conclusion of Chapter 2) to be able to make this analysis. Grice (1975) offers certain principles which should guide us in this respect.

Quantity:

1 Make your contribution as informative as possible

2. Do not make your contribution more informative than is required or your listener will be misled or think you talk too much.

Quality:

1 Do not say what you believe to be false.

2 Do not say that for which you lack adequate evidence

Relation

Manner:

1 Avoid obscurity of expression

2 Avoid ambiguity

3 Be brief

4 Be orderly.

If these rules are not observed, Grice suggests that the listener starts to seek for the implied meaning, or he looks for some context within which the speaker's message can be understood. The dysphasic person can hardly be expected to comply with these rules but it is salutory for the speech therapist to listen to her own side of the dialogue and note how often she herself fails to be clear, truthful and orderly. Such an analysis should serve more purposes than self-castigation. It should reveal just what is taking place during a verbal exchange. How much information is actually given and received? Did the conversation fulfil the purpose for which it was intended? If not where did it start to go wrong?

The applications of pragmatics of language to normal and disordered speech are discussed by Rees (1978) and there is a useful review of Bates' work in the volume of the British Journal of Disorders of Communication for the same year by Duchan. In the monograph, *Language Disorders in Children* (1979) the author is recorded in discussion with a boy of 5 years of age. They are looking at a model with movable figures which can be set to represent various domestic scenes.

Therapist: 'There's somebody else coming now. Who's this?'

J: 'Peter.'

Therapist: 'Well, what's Peter going to do?'

J: 'Coming to the little boy.'

Therapist: 'Peter's going up to the little boy. Right-ho. Now then, what is Peter going to say?'

J: 'I'm going to give you the ball.'

Therapist: 'That was lovely. And what does the little boy say?'

J: 'Yes.'

Therapist: 'Yes what?'

J: 'Yes please.'

Therapist: 'He might. Or he might say, thank you very much Peter. Do you think he might? You say it. What does he say? Do you remember what he says? What does he say?'

J: 'I shall give the ball, Peter.'

Therapist: 'That's right. And what does he say when Peter gives him the ball? What do you think he says? What does he say?'

J: 'I shall give the ball Peter.'

Therapist: 'That's right. And what does *he* say when Peter gives him the ball? What do you think he says? Is he pleased?'

J: 'Yes.'

Therapist: 'So what does he say?'

J: 'Please can I have the ball?'

Therapist: 'Yes, that's lovely.'

The child in question is known to have language difficulties and the passage quoted shows his lapses in comprehension. But what exactly is he expected to comprehend? The two are looking at representational toys and the therapist is making suggestions. The child responds with straightforward answers at first, showing he has recognised that a question is being asked and showing that he knows the appropriate language forms. He is not entirely correct in his use of the form 'coming to' but he produces a well formulated sentence subsequently. He then gives a minimal but appropriate response and when the therapist tries to extend it she gets the automatic response to the form of her question, not to the implicit statement 'yes, and what does he say then?' The therapist then starts to be encouraging but it is questionable whether she conveys to the child exactly what it is she wants him to do. Certainly she speaks too much. However persuasive her tone, the actual words used cannot convey to the child without obscurity and ambiguity, what she meant. The child picks up what clues he can and responds to isolated words rather than meaning.

We may surmise that the little boy never really gained control of the pragmatics of language during his development of form and content. When testing his comprehension therefore we should not only look at his understanding of explicit language but his comprehension of what is implied. The therapist should not take for granted that the child knows what is implied and she should not discharge the child until she has been able to assist him towards some recognition of what underlies words.

The development of language units will give increased impetus for work of this kind and many more opportunities to carry it out. Teacher and therapist can work together to devise activities which will stimulate the child to get his ideas across to other people. Verbal mastery requires some struggle by the child and then judicious help and consequent language building by those working with him. Psychologists and teachers are used to working with content and function and speech therapists with content and form and the linking of the disciplines should be fruitful. They will be very strongly needed to help those language impaired children whose first language is not English. Here we do not only encounter problems of linguistic structure but difficulties in appreciating the role of language in the child's community. As Britain becomes a multi-racial society the onus upon speech therapy services to extend their work in a socio-linguistic direction will increase. We are just starting to investigate bilingulism in relation to our own professional contribution (Miller, 1978; Abudarham, 1980) and there will be many implications to be explored if we are to offer a realistic service. The

College of Speech Therapists has recently appointed Sam Abudarham and Sian Munro to advise therapists in this area.

Increased co-operation with teachers and psychologists will stimulate many speech therapists to look at their responsibility with regard to reading. Most members of the profession have followed the lead given by the Quirk Committee (p68.6.44,45,46) and concentrated their attention on verbal language while maintaining interest in its relationship with the printed form. There is a small but strong nucleus of opinion which insists that speech therapists involve themselves in the graphic form of language as a professional duty. This opinion lead the college to appoint Bevé Hornsby and Mary Manning Thomas, both very experienced in dyslexia and allied language disorders to advise interested therapists (see also de Montfort Supple, 1980 and for normal development Perera, 1979).

We are certainly seeing a considerable increase in the number of tasks which a speech therapist now tackles and of the fields of interest with which she is occupied. The extent to which these will change her image is a matter for speculation.

It is suggested by some writers that the clinician's role is associated with value judgements and keeps the speech-handicapped child or adult in a dependent position. Forms of therapy e.g. communication therapy are accordingly devised which are focused upon self-directed activity (Buck, 1980). Doubtless such programmes are very valuable, as are many creative activities stimulated by thoughtful people, but it is not necessary to deduce that the clinical role is oppressive and didactic. It is perfectly possible for a clinician working in a medical environment to serve her patient creatively respecting his goals and drives. If the group is seen as the therapeutic vehicle the clinical model is not appropriate and the therapist will be much more helpfully employed in organising her group in the community. This kind of approach is viewed sympathetically by many present day students and young clinicians and it may extend itself. The original relationship between therapist and patient on which speech therapy practice has been based arose from the medical model. The speech therapist, modelling herself upon the doctor, offered healing skills and in return the patient offered trust. The relationship was one where confidentiality was a hallmark. Speech therapists were trained to treat all confidences with respect and not to pass on information from the patient without his consent. They were also trained to protect medical information. These ethics are still proper and necessary and this generation of students can accept them without difficulty. What they are unable to accept nearly so easily is the middle class professional role. Present day students have been brought up amid a much more sociologically influenced clime and have been trained to experiment with roles rather then accept them unquestioningly. Nevertheless the figure of the sympathetic and skilful therapist with access to medical information has a great deal to offer troubled people. Parents can be helped as much within an individual treatment session for a child as by a group discussion. They are often and very reasonably looking for authority and expertise in an area where they feel confused and ignorant.

Speech therapists have always worked with parents and it has been an individual decision as to whether the therapist leads and the mother supports or vice versa. Sometimes, as in the case of Secundus, described in Chapter 7 the therapist will take over the mother's role in language until she is able to take it up again. Sometimes she advises the mother and takes little active part in the therapy (Clezy, 1979). The involvement of parents in all aspects of their handicapped children's progress is now a dominant educational and medical feature and all future speech therapists must accept this collaboration. It is not always easy. By the time a parent comes to the speech therapist she may have a great deal of stored up anger to work through. In reviewing the account by Elizabeth Browning of the medical and educational history of her aphasic son (1973) the author commented upon the need of parents 'to speak back to the experts who appear to pronounce upon them so cursorily; and perhaps above all to pay some kind of tribute to the special quality of their handicapped child whose spirit can only be revealed to those who see him in his daily frustrations and humiliations and in his daily pleasures and small, life enhancing achievements.' The review concludes by commending the book which 'offers the mature reader the opportunity to percieve his true role in the difficult but essential dialogue between those who suffer and those who try to heal'.

Mrs Browning, in her work as chairman of AFASIC, a parent based association started by a speech therapist, has done much to assist parents of speech handicapped children. Similar work has been done by Diana Law, herself the victim of aphasia, in helping the adult. There are now therefore a number of voluntary bodies with whom the College of Speech Therapists is in steady and active consultation and these include speech handicapped persons, their relatives and volunteers who wish to help in the work. The prospective therapist must embrace this relationship also and see it as her role to work with volunteers in the service of the speech handicapped (Goodwins 1980). She may prepare for this by attending stroke and speech clubs while in training or by taking part in the AFASIC holiday scheme. Or she may carry out her supervised practice as a student in conditions where volunteers are involved in assisting the speech therapist. There is every reason to believe that the protective isolation believed to be enjoyed by the medically based therapist is now at an end. In fact the present movement is the logical development of moves already taken by individual clinicians but it is none the worse for that.

Whatever else the present and future activities of the speech therapist do they must certainly dispel the out-moded idea that patients are invariably given specific treatment at half-hourly intervals at the speech clinic. Speech therapists must be allowed a new range of flexibility in the way they apportion their time if they are to be able to make use of their skills and knowledge to the best advantage of the patient. It is up to the new generation of speech therapists to maintain the drive exerted by the present protagonists towards this end. They will have been trained to take more account of ideas in other disciplines and must continue to do so. This intellectual widening will also allow the new therapist to capitalise much more quickly upon research activities. She will be able to involve herself in medical findings far more actively than her predecessors have been. She has better access to university laboratories and is better trained scientifically. Because she has been trained to some extent in research methodology she will be able to appreciate research findings in medical areas. This is likely to be very important as we receive more information on the nature of brain function and other aspects of neurological organisation. As has been repeatedly stressed in these chapters, most of the hard core speech and language handicaps are those which have an undiscovered but suspected neurological basis. All the group of conditions discussed under developmental aphasia and apraxia are showing symptoms of neurological failure which we cannot help patients transcend because we can only see, very dimly what they are up against.

Our treatment methods are still very crude and need refinement by better understanding of neurophysiological function. The present day student is likely to receive her training in institutions which are actively engaged in research. This is probably the major difference between present and past training. It will be assumed that research into conditions affecting language is going on and students will equip themselves to make use of the findings. They will thus be in a better position to make immediate therapeutic capital out of medical and scientific research than those of us who had to be patiently trained in the language and the method before we could start to read introductory literature. This is hardly to state that neurophysiological research can be understood by a speech therapy student any more than it can by a medical student or a student of psychology, but the expectation will be that problems have solutions. The speech therapy student can at least develop a research attitude and read at the level of the more general scientific and medical investigations. Thus she will be prepared to take further moves forward as they become possible. Many conditions now are waiting upon neurophysiological and biochemical discoveries and when these are made we want to be able to take advantage of them just as we have of those of physics in our use of equipment and linguistic analysis in our assessments.

We may also hope to get better as a profession, in asking the right questions to stimulate research. In the past the gap between what we observed as clinicians and what we could define for purposes of experiment, was much too wide. More minute and scientifically controlled observation by speech therapists together with more understanding by them of the approaches and limits of research may produce a more productive meeting.

Finally it seems that speech therapy students are indeed in a fortunate position with so much opportunity and so much on which to build. Only less fortunate perhaps than those of us now in middle age who have seen our profession emerge under its own banner and can still contemplate enthusiastically the discoveries that lie ahead.

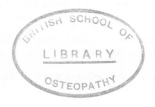

References

SECTION 1
Preface
Quirk R (Chairman) 1972 Speech therapy services. Report of the Committee of Enquiry. HMSO, London

Chapter 2
Cooper J, Moodley M, Reynell J 1978 Helping language development. Edward Arnold, London
Griffiths C P S 1972 Developmental dysphasia an introduction. Invalid Children's Aid Assn., London
Reynell J 1969 Reynell developmental language scales. N F E R Slough, Bucks

Further reading
Polanyi M 1971 Tacit knowing: In: Knowing and being. Routledge Kegan Paul, London

Chapter 3
Boston diagnostic aphasia examination 1976 Kimpson London
Butfield E 1958 Rehabilitation of the dysphasic patient. Speech Pathology and Therapy 1(1)
Byers Brown B 1971 Speak for yourself. Educational Explorers, Reading
Byers Brown B, Ives L 1969 The re-education of a dysphasic adult: an experiment in co-operation between a speech therapist and an educational psychologist. British Journal of Disorders of Communication 4(2): 176–196
Cruse D A 1978 A case of auditory subseption in an adult aphasic (unpublished)
Edwards M 1973 Developmental verbal dyspraxia. British Journal of Disorders of Communication 8(1): 64–70
Eisenson J 1954 Examining for aphasia. The Psychological Corp, New York
Garvey M, Kellet B 1975 Case studies of three 'xxyy' children. British Journal of Disorders of Communication 10(1): 17–30
Greene M C L 1963 A comparison of children with delayed speech due to co-ordination disorder or language learning difficulty. Speech Pathology and Therapy 6:69.
Morley M 1972 Development and disorders of speech in childhood, 3rd edn. Churchill Livingstone, Edinburgh
Minnesota test for differential diagnosis 1965 University of Minnesota Press, Minneapolis
Trim J L M 1967 A Linguistic review of a case of dysphasia. Department of Audiology and Education of the Deaf, University of Manchester

Chapter 4
Byers Brown B, Beveridge M (ed) 1979 Language disorders in children. A Workshop for Teachers. College of Speech Therapists, London

Cruttenden A 1979 Language in infancy and childhood. University Press, Manchester

Greene M C L 1972 The voice and its disorders, 3rd edn. Pitman Medical, London

Jeffree D M, McConkey R 1976 Let me speak. Souvenir Press, London

McConkey R, Jeffree D M and Hewson S 1979 Involving parents in extending the language development of their young mentally handicapped children. British Journal of Disorders of Communication 14(3): 203–218

McCartney, Byers Brown B 1980 A speech teaching scheme for A T C instructions. British Journal of Disorders of Communication 15(2)

Chapter 5

Court D 1976 (Chairman) Fit for the future. Report of the Committee of Enquiry into Child Health Services H M S O, London

Fry D 1978 Home Loquens. University Press, Cambridge

Lea J 1970 The colour pattern scheme. A method of remedial teaching. Moor House School, Oxted

McCartney E 1979 The construction of audio-visual programme of language training for the use of staff in adult training centres. Unpublished M Ed thesis, University of Manchester

McCartney E, Byers Brown B 1980 Instructor participation in a speech therapy programme for adult trainees. The British Journal of Mental Subnormality (in press)

Warnock M 1978 (Chairman) Special education needs. Report of the Committee of Enquiry into the Education of Handicapped Children and Young People HMSO, London

Whelan E, Speake B 1977 Adult training centres in England and Wales. National Association of Teachers of the Mentally Handicapped

Further reading

Bliss C K 1965 Semantography. Semantography Publications, Sydney Australia

Fawcus R 1979 Official aids for the disabled conference and exhibition. In: Bulletin of the College of Speech Therapists 333 January 1980

Health Equipment Information 1980 D H S S 83

Lyle L L 1976 Communication assessment and intervention strategies. University Park Press, Baltimore

Paget R, Gorman P 1968 A systematic sign language. NID, London

Skelly M Amerind gestural code (based on universal hand talk.) Thonono Books, Limerick, Ireland

Walker M 1976 The revised Makaton vocabulary. Bottings Park Hospital, Chertsey, Surrey

Chapter 6

Byers Brown B 1974 some aspects of delayed speech. Unpublished M Ed thesis, University of Manchester

College of Speech Therapists 1970 Evidence submitted to the Committee of Enquiry into Speech Therapy Services

Cruttenden A 1979 Language in infancy and childhood. University Press, Manchester

Dalton P, Hardcastle W 1977 Disorders of fluency. Studies in Language Disability and Remediation 3

Eisenson J 1968 Developmental aphasia: a speculative view with therapeutic implications. Journal of Speech and Hearing Disorders 33(1): 3–13

Ewing A W G 1930 Aphasia in children. Oxford University Press, London

Grady P A E 1963 Towards a new concept of dyslalia In: signs symbols and signals. Methuen, London p 159–165

Grunwell P 1975 The phonological analysis of articulation disorders. British Journal of Disorders of Communication 10(1): 31–42

Halpern H 1972 Adult aphasia. The Bobbs Merrill Company Inc Indianapolis, New York

Ingram T T S 1972 The classification of speech and language disorders in young children. In: Rutter and Bax (ed) The child with delayed speech. Heineman Medical, London, p 13–32

Kracke I 1975 Perception of rhythmic sequences by aphasic and deaf children. British Journal of Disorders of Communication 10(1): 43–51

Laver J D M 1968 Voice quality and indexical information. British Journal of Disorders of Communication 3(1): 43–54

Luchsinger R, Arnold G 1965 Voice speech and language. Wadsworth Belmont, Calif

Morley M 1972 Development and disorders of speech in childhood, 3rd edn. Churchill Livingstone, Edinburgh

Mysak E D 1976 Pathologies of speech systems. Williams and Wilkins Co, Baltimore

Smith N V 1974 The acquistion of phonological skills in children. British Journal of Disorders of Communication 9(1): 17–23

Tallal P, Piercy M 1978 Defects of auditory perception in children with developmental dysphasia. In : Wyke (ed) Developmental dysphasia, p 63–84

Van Riper C, Irwin J V 1958 Voice and articulation. Pitman Medical, London

Warnock M (Chairman) 1978 Special educational needs. Report of the Committee of Enquiry into the Education of Handicapped Children and Young People

Wood K S 1971 Terminology and nomenclature In: Travis (ed) Handbook of speech pathology and audiology. Appleton Century Crofts, New York

Wyke B 1969 Deus machina vocis. An analysis of the laryngeal reflex mechanisms of speech. British Journal of Disorders of Communication 4(1): 3–25

Wynter H 1974 An investigation into the analysis and terminology of voice quality. British Journal of Disorders of Communication 9(2): 102–110

Zangwill O L 1978 The concept of developmental dysphasia In: Wyke (ed) Developmental dysphasia. Academic Press, London New York

Further reading

Haas, W 1963 Phonological analysis of a case of dyslalia. Journal of Speech and Hearing Disorders 28(3)

Rockey D 1963 some fundamental principles for the solution of terminological problem in speech pathology. British Journal of Disorders of Communications 4(2) 160–175

SECTION II
Chapter 7

Aitchison J 1972 Mini malapropisms. British Journal of Disorders of Communication

Bangs J 1942 A clinical analysis of the articulatory defects of the feeble minded. Journal of Speech Disorders 7: 343–356

Benton A 1978 The cognitive functioning of children with developmental dysphasia. In: Wyke (ed) Developmental dysphasia. Academic Press, London, p 43–62

Berry M F, Eisenson J 1956 Speech disorders. Appleton Century Crofts, New York

Bloom L, Lahey M 1978 Language development and language disorders. John Wiley and Sons, London

Bobath K B 1976 Motor development in the different types of cerebral palsy. Heineman, London

Crickmay M 1966 Speech therapy and the Bobath approach to cerebral palsy. Springfield, Illinois

Byers Brown 1966 The facilitation of speech in children with mental and motor retardation. Proceedings of the Chicago Conference of the American Association of Mental Retardation, Chicago

Byers Brown 1972 An attempt to facilitate the acquisition of language in a four year old child. A I L A Proceedings, Copenhagen

Byers Brown 1977 Address to conference of heads of schools for the deaf. Department of Audiology and Education of the Deaf University of Manchester

Carlson E 1941 Born that way. John Day Co, New York

Cooper J, Moodley M and Reynell J 1978 Helping language development. Edward Arnold, London

Cotton E 1965 The institute of movement therapy and school for conductors. A report on a study visit. Developmental Medicine and Child Neurology 7(4): 437–46

Crystal D 1979 Working with LARSP. Edward Arnold, London

Doman Delacato see Delacato C H 1963 The diagnosis and treatment of speech and reading problems. Charles C Thomas, Springfield, Illinois

Ewing A W G 1930 Aphasia in children. Oxford University Press, London

Freeman R D 1967 Controversy over 'patterning' as a treatment for brain damage in children. Journal of the American Medical Association 202(5): 385–388

Fry D 1977 Address to conference of heads of schools for the deaf. Department of Audiology and Education of the Deaf University of Manchester

Fry D 1978 Homo loquens. Cambridge University Press.

Grimley A, McKinlay I 1977 The clumsy child. Assn. of Pediatric Chartered Physiotherapists Crawley, Sussex

Jeffree D M, MConkey R 1976 Let me speak souvenir Press London

King A, Parker A 1980 The relevance of prosodic features to speech work with hearing impaired children. In: Jones F M (ed) Language disability in children. M T P, Lancaster

Kracke I 1975 Perception of rhythmic sequences by aphasic and deaf children. British Journal of Disorders of Communication 10(1): 43–51

Markides A 1970 The speech of deaf and partially hearing children with special reference to factors affecting intelligibility. British Journal of Disorders of Communication 5(2)

Matthews J 1971 Communication disorders in the mentally retarded In: Travis (ed) Handbook of Speech Pathology and Audiology 31: 801–818

McGinnis M 1963 Aphasic children. Alexander Graham Bell Assn., Washington DC

Morley M C 1973 Receptive expressive developmental aphasia. British Journal of Disorders of Communication 8(1): 47–53

Mentally handicapped children: A plan for action, DHSS, London

National Development Group for the Mentally Handicapped 2 1977

Reeds D M, Wing L 1976 Language communication and the use of symbols. In: Wing (ed) Early childhood autism.

Renfrew C E 1966 Persistence of the open syllable in defective articulation Journal of Speech and Hearing Disorders 31: 370–73

Rutter M Concepts of autism. A review of the literature. Journal of Child Psychology and Psychiatry 9: 1–25

Rutter M (ed) 1971 Infantile autism. Churchill Livingstone, Edinburgh London

Strauss A A, Lehtinen C E 1947 Psychopathology and education of the brain injured child. Greene and Stratton, New York

Taylor I G 1966 Hearing in relation to language disorders in children. British Journal of Disorders of Communication 1(1): 11–20

Van Riper C, Irwin J V 1968 Voice and articulation. Pitman Medical Press, London

Walton J N, Ellis E and Court S D M 1962 Clumsy children. A study of developmental dyspraxia. Brain 85

Warner J 1980 Helping your handicapped child with early feeding. A manual for parents. University of Manchester

Further reading
Cruickshank W (ed) Cerebral palsy, 3rd edn. Syracuse University Press, New York
Ward S, McCarthy E Congenital auditory imperception. A follow-up study. British
    Journal of disorders of Communication 13(1): 3–16

Chapter 8
Crystal D, Fletcher P and Garman M 1976 The grammatical analysis of language
    disability. Studies in language disability and remediation 1. Edward Arnold,
    London
Curtiss S 1977 Genie a psycho-linguistic study of a modern day 'wild child.'
    Academic Press, London
Ingram T T S, Anthony A, Bogle D, McIsaac M W 1971 The Edinburgh
    articulation test. Churchill Livingstone, Edinburgh
Ingram D 1976 Phonological disability in children. Studies in language disability
    and remediation 2. Edward Arnold, London
Menyuk P 1978 Linguistic problems in children with developmental dysphasia In:
    Wyke (ed) Developmental dysphasia. Academic Press, London, p 135–158
Muma J R 1978 Language handbook concepts assessment intervention.
    Prentice-Hall Englewood Cliffs, New Jersey
Mussen P H, Conger J I and Kagan J Child development and personality, 4th edn.
    Harpers International Edition. Harper & Row, London
Williams D 1971 Stuttering therapy for children In: Travis (ed) Handbook of speech
    pathology and audiology 41: 1073–1093

Further reading
Berry M 1969 Language disorders of children. Appleton Century Crofts, New York

Chapter 9
Ballard C F, Bond E K 1960 Clinical observations between variations of jaw form
    and variations of oro-facial behaviour including those for articulation. Speech
    Pathology and Therapy 3(2): 55–63
Byers Brown B, Beveridge M (ed) 1979 Language disorders in children a workshop
    for teachers. College of Speech Therapists, London
Butler N R, Peckham C S and Sheridan M D 1973 Speech defects in children aged
    7 years. British Medical Journal 1: 253
Compton A J 1976 Generative studies of children's phonological disorders: clinical
    ramifications In: Morehead and Morehead (ed) Normal and deficient child
    language. University Park Press, Baltimore London
Connor P Stork F C 1972 Linguistics and speech therapy a case study. British
    Journal of Disorders of Communication 7(1): 44–48
Cooper J M, Griffiths P 1978 Treatment and prognosis. In: Wyke (ed)
    Developmental dysphasia. Academic Press, London p 159–176
Cruttenden A 1972 Phonological procedures for child language. British Journal of
    Disorders of Communication 7(1): 30–37
Dalton, P, Hardcastle W J 1977 Disorders of fluency 3. Studies in language
    disability and remediation. Edward Arnold, London
Fawcus R 1980 The treatment of phonological disorders In: Jones M F (ed)
    Language disability in children. MTP, Lancaster, p 159–177
Grady PAE 1973 Language and the pre-school child. British Journal of Disorders of
    Communication 8(1): 42–46
Grunwell P 1975 The phonological analysis of articulation disorders. British Journal
    of Disorders of Communication 10(1): 31–42
Grunwell P 1980 Developmental language disorders at the phonological level In:
    Jones M F (ed) Language disability in children. MTP, Lancaster, p 129–158
Gwynne Evans E 1972 The biological destiny of the oro-facial muscles. British
    Journal of Disorders of Communication 7(2): 110–116

Ingram D 1976 Phonological disability in children. Studies in language disability and remediation 2. Edward Arnold, London

Irwin J V 1972 Disorders of articulation. The Bobbs-Merrill Company Inc, Indianapolis New York

Lapointe C 1976 Token test performances by learning disabled and achieving adolescents. British Journal of Disorders of Communication 11(2): 121–133

McGinnis M A 1963 Aphasic children. Alexander Graham Bell Assn, Washington DC

Peckham C S 1973 Speech defects in a national sample of children aged 7 years. British Journal of Disorders of Communication 8(1): 2–8

Powers M Hall 1971 Clinical and educational procedures in functional disorders of articulation. In: Travis (ed) Handbook of Speech Pathology and Audiology 34: 877–910

Renfrew C E, Geary L 1973 Prediction of persisting speech defect. British Journal of Disorders of Communication 8(1): 37–41

Sheridan M D 1973 Children of 7 years with marked speech defects. British Journal of Disorders of Communication 8(1): 9–16

Siegel Broen 1976 Language assessment. In: Lloyd L (ed) Communication assessment and intervention strategies. University Park Press, Baltimore, p 73–122

Smith N V 1973 The acquisition of phonology a case study. University Press, Cambridge

Van Thal J 1954 Tongue thrust in relation to sigmatism. Speech 18(1): 24–26

Warnock M (Chairman) 1978 Special educational needs. Report of the committee of enquiry into the education of handicapped children and young people

Wiig E H 1976 Language disabilities of adolescents. British Journal of Disorders of Communication 11(1): 3–17

Wiig E H, Semel E M 1976 Language disabilities in children and adolescents. Charles E Merrill, Columbus Ohio

Winitz H 1969 Articulatory acquisition and behaviour. Appleton Century Crofts, New York

Chapter 10

Arnold C E 1960 Studies in tachyphemia 1 and 3. Logos 3(1) and (2)

Barlow W 1973 The Alexander principle. Victor Gollancz, London

Boomer D S, Laver J D M 1968 Slips of the tongue. British Journal of Disorders of Communication 3(1): 2–12

*Boone Daniel R The voice and voice therapy. Prentice-Hall, Englewood Cliffs New Jersey

Bull T, Cook Joyce 1976 Speech therapy and ENT surgery. Blackwell's Scientific Publications, Oxford

*Dalton P, Hardcastle W J 1977 Disorders of fluency. Studies in language disability and remediation 3

Fitch D B 1963 The assessment of defective speech in an adult In: signs signals and symbols. Methuen London p 175–182

Gordon M T 1975 The value of aerodynamic analysis in the treatment of dysphonia. Proceedings of 7th National Conference 231–241 College of Speech Therapists, London

*Green M C L 1972 The voice and its disorders, 3rd edn. Pitman Medical, London

Jacobson E 1938 Progressive relaxation. University Press, Chicago

Kelman A W 1975 The application of aerodynamic studies of voice pathology proceedings of the 7th National Conference 215–230 College of Speech Therapists, London

Laver J D M 1968 Voice quality and indexical information. British Journal of Disorders of Communication 3(1): 43–54

Luchsinger R, Arnold G 1965 Voice – speech – language. Wadsworth Belmont, Calif
Nauta Walle J H, Feirtag M 1979 The organisation of the brain. Scientific American 241(3)
Simpson I C 1971 Dysphonia: the organisation and working of a dysphonia clinic. British Journal of Disorders of Communication 6(1): 70–85
Simpson I C 1975 The future of voice pathology. Proceedings of 7th National Conference College of Speech Therapists, London
Weiss D A 1964 Cluttering. Prentice-Hall, Engleford Cliffs, New York
Wohl M T 1968 The electronic metronome – an evaluative study. British Journal of Disorders of Communication 3(1): 89–98
Wynter H 1974 An investigation into the analysis and terminology of voice quality. British Journal of Disorders of Communication 9(2): 102–110

Further reading
Fink B 1975 The human larynx. Raven Press, New York
Gregory H H (ed) 1979 Controversies about stuttering therapy. University Park Press, Baltimore
Travis L E (ed) 1971 Handbook of Speech Pathology and Audiology Part 3 Voice 441–505 and Part 4 Speech 995–1109
Van Riper C 1971 The nature of stuttering. Prentice-Hall Englewood Cliffs, New York

See also full texts of the works indicated with asterisk.

Chapter 11
Allan C M 1970 Treatment of non-fluent speech resulting from neurological disease. British Journal of Disorders of Communication 5(1): 3–5
Butfield E 1952 An introduction to the assessment of aphasia patients. Speech (2)
Butfield E 1961 Speech therapy and acquired dysarthria. Speech Pathology and Therapy 4(2): 74–80
Byers Brown B, Ives L 1969 The re-education of a dysphasic adult: an experiment in co-operation between a speech therapist and an educational psychologist. British Journal of Disorders of Communication 4(2): 176–196
Byers Brown B 1971 Speak for yourself. Educational Explorers, Reading
Cruse D A 1978 A case of auditory subception in an adult aphasic (unpublished)
Darley F L 1972 The efficacy of language rehabilitation in aphasia. Journal of Speech and Hearing Disorders 37(1): 3–21
Darley F L, Aronson A E, Brown 1975 Motor speech disorders. W B Saunders and Co, London
Enderby P 1979 Frenchay dysarthria assessment. Frenchay, Bristol
Fitch B 1957 The value of bi-weekly speech therapy for adults with acquired aphasia. Unpublished MCST thesis of College of Speech Therapists
Geschwind N 1965 Disconnection syndrome in animals and man. Brain 88: 237–294: 585–644
Goodglass H, Kaplan E 1976 The assessment of aphasia and related disorders. Henry Kimpton, London
Halpern H 1972 Adult aphasia. Bobbs-Merrill Company Inc., Indianapolis
Hatfield F M 1972 Looking for help from linguistics: an approach to aphasic problems. British Journal of Disorders of Communication 7(1): 64–82
Langley J, Darvill G 1979 PNF A practical manual. c/o C.S.T., London
Lesser R 1978 Linguistic investigations of aphasia. Studies in language disability and remediation 4. Edward Arnold, London
Lott B 1979 Dysarthria – a case study. Journal of the International Phonetic Association 9(1)
Luria A R 1966 Higher cortical functions in man. Basic Books, New York

Luria A R 1970 The functional organisation of the brain. Scientific American 222 March p 66

Porch B 1967 The Porch index of communicative ability. Consulting Psychological Press, Palo Alto

Sarno M T, Silver M A M, Sands E 1970 Speech therapy and language recovery in severe aphasia. Journal of Speech and Hearing Disorders 13: 607–623

Schuell H 1965 The Minnesota test for differential diagnosis of aphasia. University of Minnesota Press, Minneapolis

Snidecor J C 1974 Speech re-habilitation of the laryngectomized, 2nd edn. Charles C Thomas Springfield, Illinois

Skelly M 1973 Glossectomee speech rehabilitation. Charles Thomas Springfield, Illinois

Sparks R, Helm N, Albert M 1974 Aphasia rehabilitation resulting from melodic intonation therapy. Cortex 10: 303–316

Wepman J M, Jones L V 1961 Language modalities test for aphasia. Education Industry Service Chicago

Further reading

Brown J 1972 Aphasia apraxia and agnosia. Charles C Thomas, Springfield, Illinois

Brown J 1977 Mind brain and consciousness. Academic Press, London

Eisenson J 1971 Aphasia in adults. In: Travis (op. cit)

Jenkins J J, Pabon E, Shaw R, Sefer J 1975 Schuell's aphasia in adults, 2nd edn. Harper and Row, London

Outcome of severe damage to the central nervous system 1975. CIBA Foundation Symposium, 34

Travis L E (ed) 1971 Handbook of Speech Pathology and Audiology Part 3 Voice 571–616

See also bibliographies listed in Halpern and Lesser

Chapter 12

Abudarham S 1980 The problems of the linguistic potential of children with dual language systems and their implications for the formulation of a differential diagnosis In: Jones M F (ed) Language disability in children. MTD, Lancaster p 231–244

Bates E 1976 Pragmatics and sociolinguistics in child language In: Morehead and Morehead (eds) Normal and deficient child language. University Park Press, Baltimore, p 411–468

Bates E 1978 Language and context. The acquisition of pragmatics. Academic Press, New York

Broadbent D E 1971 Introduction. Cognitive psychology. British Medical Bulletin 27(3): 191–194

Byers Brown 1972 Reviewing the above. British Disorders of Communication 7(1): 98–99

Browning E 1973 I can't see what you are saying. Paul Elek, London

Byers Brown B 1973 Reviewing the above. British Journal of Disorders of Communication 8(1): 80–81

Buck L A 1980 Dynamics of communication disorders in a hearing and speech centre In: Jones M F (ed) Language Disability in children MTP, Lancaster p 95–109

Byers Brown B, Beveridge M (eds) 1979 Language disorders in children. CST London

Clezy G 1978 Modification of the mother-child interchange in language speech and hearing. University Park Press, Baltimore

Clezy G 1978 Modification of the mother-child interchange. British Journal of Disorders of Communication 13(2): 93–106

Grice H P 1975 Logic and Conversation In: Cole P, Morgan J L (eds) Syntax and semantics 3. Speech acts. Academic Press, New York

Halliday M A K 1975 Learning how to mean – explorations in language study. Edward Arnold, London

Miller N 1978 The bi-lingual child in the speech clinic. British Journal of Disorders of Communication 13(1): 17–30

de Montford Supple Sister Marie 1980 Reading as one aspect of language In: Jones F (ed) Language disability in children. MTP, Lancaster p 111–128

Perera K 1979 Reading and writing In: Cruttenden A Language in infancy and childhood. University of Manchester p 130–160

Further reading

AFASIC 1973 Holiday project 1973. Association for all speech impaired children, London

Beveridge M, Lloyd P 1977 The developing person as communicator. Paper given at the Annual Conference of the British Psychological Society Development Section. Cambridge.

Goodwins R 1980 Unpublished address to College of Speech Therapists and VOCAL association of voluntary bodies

Rees N 1978 I don't understand what you mean by comprehension. Journal of Speech and Hearing Disorders 42: 208–219

Glossary

ABBREVIATIONS AND SPECIAL TERMS

AFASIC	Association For All Speech Impaired Children
ATC	Adult Training Centre
CAT	computerized axial tomography
CVA	cerebrovascular accident
DAF	delayed auditory feedback
EMI scan	technique developed from the apparatus designed by EMI now known as CAT scan
ENT	ear, nose and throat
ESN(M)	educationally sub-normal (mild)
ESN(S)	educationally sub-normal (severe)
GP	General Practitioner
HF	high frequency
Hz	Hertz or cycles per second
ITPA	Illinois test of Psycholinguistic Abilities
LARSP	Language Assessment, Remediation and Screening Procedure
NCB	National Children's Bureau
PNF	Proprioceptive Neuromuscular Facilitation
WISC	Wechsler Intelligence Scale for Children

COMMUNICATION AIDS

SPLINK Speech Link
POSSUM Patient Operated Selector Mechanism

Special terms referring to non-verbal communication systems are given in the references. Not all the items of equipment mentioned in Chapter 5 are referenced for reasons which are implicit in the whole chapter. The following texts may be studied to illustrate the use of:

Nasendoscopy and nasal anemometry

Ellis R E, Flack F C (eds) Diagnosis and treatment of palato glossal malfunction. The College of Speech Therapists Monograph No. 2 (1979) in association with the British Journal of Disorders of Communication.

The Edinburgh masker

Dewar A, Dewar A D, Anthony J F K The effect of auditory feedback masking on concomitant movements of stammering. British Journal of Disorders of Communication vol 11, no 2, October, 1976, p 95–102

Dewar A, Dewar A D, Barnes H E Automatic triggering of auditory feedback masking in stammering and cluttering. The British Journal of Disorders of Communication vol 11, no. 1, 1976

The relaxometer

Rustin L An intensive programme for adolescent stammerers. The British Journal of Disorders of Communication vol 13, no. 2 October, 1978, p 85–92

The voiscope

Wirz S L, Anthony J The use of the voiscope in improving the speech of profoundly deaf children. The British Journal of Disorders of Communication vol 14, no. 2 1980

SPEECH THERAPY SERVICES

At the time of going to press the speech therapy team is headed by the Area Speech Therapist. She is supported by Chief Speech Therapists and Senior Speech Therapists at general or specialized grades. As this structure is under review other titles may appear in the future. Confusion can be avoided if readers take note of the present hierarchy and substitute forthcoming titles as appropriate.

Subject Index